ABC of
Clinical Professionalism

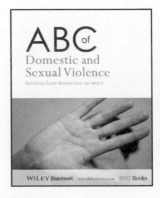
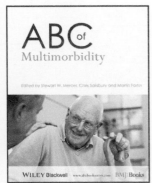
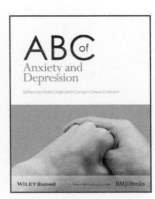
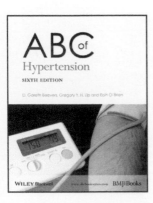

ABC of
Clinical
Professionalism

EDITED BY

Nicola Cooper
Derby Teaching Hospitals and University of Nottingham
UK

Anna Frain
University of Nottingham
UK

John Frain
University of Nottingham
UK

WILEY Blackwell

This edition first published 2018 © 2018 by John Wiley & Sons Ltd.

The right of Nicola Cooper, Anna Frain and John Frain to be identified as the author(s) of the editorial material in this work has been asserted in accordance with law.

Registered Office(s)
John Wiley & Sons, Inc., 111 River Street, Hoboken, NJ 07030, USA
John Wiley & Sons Ltd, The Atrium, Southern Gate, Chichester, West Sussex, PO19 8SQ, UK

Editorial Office
9600 Garsington Road, Oxford, OX4 2DQ, UK

For details of our global editorial offices, customer services, and more information about Wiley products visit us at www.wiley.com.

Wiley also publishes its books in a variety of electronic formats and by print-on-demand. Some content that appears in standard print versions of this book may not be available in other formats.

Library of Congress Cataloging-in-Publication Data
Names: Cooper, Nicola, editor. | Frain, Anna, editor. | Frain, John (John
    Patrick James), editor.
Title: ABC of clinical professionalism / [edited] by Nicola Cooper, Anna
    Frain, John Frain.
Description: Hoboken, NJ : Wiley, 2017. | Series: ABC series | Includes
    bibliographical references and index. |
Identifiers: LCCN 2017033964 (print) | LCCN 2017035045 (ebook) | ISBN
    9781119266686 (pdf) | ISBN 9781119266693 (epub) | ISBN 9781119266662
    (paper)
Subjects: | MESH: Professionalism | Patient Care–ethics | Confidentiality |
    Leadership
Classification: LCC R118 (ebook) | LCC R118 (print) | NLM W 50 | DDC 610–dc23 LC record available at https://lccn.loc.gov/2017033964

Cover Design: Wiley
Cover image: Courtesy of Nicola Cooper via world.net

Set in 9.25/12pt MinionPro by SPi Global, Chennai, India

10 9 8 7 6 5 4 3 2 1

Contents

Contributors

John Alcolado DM, BM(Hons), FRCP

Division of Medical Sciences and Graduate Entry Medicine, University of Nottingham, UK

Nicola Cooper MBChB, FAcadMEd, FRCPE, FRACP

Derby Teaching Hospitals NHS Foundation Trust and Division of Graduate Entry Medicine, University of Nottingham, UK

Anna Frain MBChB, MRCGP, PGCert (Med Ed)

Division of Health Sciences and Graduate Entry Medicine, University of Nottingham, UK

John Frain MBChB, MSc, FRCGP, DGM, DCH, DRCOG, PgDipCard

Division of Medical Sciences and Graduate Entry Medicine, University of Nottingham, UK

Clare Gerada MBE, FRCGP, FRCPsych

Medical Director Practitioner Health Programme, Riverside Medical Centre, London, UK

Alison Greig BHK, BSc (PT), PhD

Department of Physical Therapy, University of British Columbia, Canada

Judy McKimm MBA, MA(Ed), BA(Hons), PGDip(HSW), SFHEA, FAcadMed

Swansea University Medical School, Swansea University, UK

John McLachlan PhD

School of Medicine, Pharmacy and Health, Durham University, Durham, UK

Lynn V. Monrouxe PhD, CPsychol, FAcadMEd

Chang Gung Medical Education Research Center (CG-MERC), Chang Gung Memorial Hospital, Linkou, Taiwan

Sue Murphy BHSc (PT), Med

Department of Physical Therapy, University of British Columbia, Canada

Andrew Papanikitas MBBS, BSc(Hons), MA(Lond), DCH, DHMSA, DPMSA, PhD

Nuffield Department of Primary Care Health Sciences, University of Oxford, UK

Charlotte E. Rees PhD, CPsychol, FHEA, FRCP(Edin)

Faculty of Medicine, Nursing and Health Sciences, Monash University, Australia

Kathryn A. Robertson BSc, MSc, MBBS

Northern Deanery, Durham University, Durham, UK

John Spandorfer MD

Jefferson Medical College, Philadelphia, USA

Clare Sutherland RGN, RN (Child), Dip MSc

Derby Teaching Hospitals NHS Foundation Trust, Derby, UK

Jill Thistlethwaite BSc, MBBS, PhD, MMEd, FRCGP, FRACGP, FHEA

University of Technology Sydney and School of Education, University of Queensland, Australia

Andy Wearn MBChB, MMedSc, MRCGP

Clinical Skills Centre, Faculty of Medicine and Health Sciences, The University of Auckland, New Zealand

Preface

Too often in describing the human condition we emphasise only the negative, dwelling at length on the lapses made by each of us. However, it is our human condition that also inspires us to acquire knowledge, to study and to collaborate in order to provide healthcare for others. We can all expect to be patients at some time in our lives. Clinical professionalism is rooted in understanding this and in empathising with our patients in the manner of our conduct, our application of knowledge and skills, and our ability to self-care and maintain our resilience.

Clinical professionalism is about the relationship between individual practitioners and patients, but also within and between teams, healthcare providers and professional bodies. Medical knowledge and technological resources have never been greater. The patient safety movement and human factors training support professionals in providing patients with ever- improving standards of healthcare. At the same time, rates of burnout and even suicide are rising among healthcare workers. The healthcare professional is also a person who requires the support of patients, colleagues and organisations in ensuring personal and professional well-being. Ultimately, this is about safe patient care.

This book is intended as an introduction to clinical professionalism for healthcare students and practitioners, a summary of the evidence currently available and an outline of a possible course on professional values in healthcare. The topics covered, while not exhaustive, reflect those of our own clinical practice in the UK's National Health Service, as well as the requirements of our own students.

Issues of clinical professionalism are strikingly similar the world over, and while local situations benefit from local solutions it has been helpful to converse with colleagues internationally and to gain a global perspective on the challenges for clinical professionalism in our time. This book has emerged from those conversations. We are immensely grateful to have had the participation of so many experts in this field – clinicians, researchers, teachers – from so many countries.

Nicola Cooper, Anna Frain and John Frain
April 2017

CHAPTER 1

Why Clinical Professionalism Matters

John Frain

Division of Medical Sciences and Graduate Entry Medicine, University of Nottingham, UK

OVERVIEW

- Clinical professionalism is founded on respect for the dignity of each human person.
- Each health professional, health service provider, professional body and regulator should 'first, do no harm' to those in their care.
- Modern professionalism is a partnership of patient and professional in an organisational framework that supports the safety and well-being of both parties.
- A duty of care acts to protect patients from a potentially unequal relationship with healthcare providers and professionals.
- A culture of rudeness and incivility in healthcare fosters cynicism and burnout in healthcare professionals and damages patient care.
- Clinical professionalism underpins safe patient care and addresses the human factors that contribute to clinical errors.

Introduction

We are all human beings. We share the same human condition – we suffer, make mistakes, we fall away from our ideals. Equally, we are all capable of greatness, of excellence and of placing the needs of others above ourselves. Each of us is unique and has a value which can never be ignored or taken away. Our roles in life should not only occupy our time but engage and bring us satisfaction. The ancient Greeks defined true happiness as the full use of one's powers along lines of excellence (see Box 1.1). These concepts have been espoused from ancient times.

We collaborate in communities and societies because it is in our interest and that of our group, because there is a mutual benefit in doing so. Some of us seek to alleviate suffering, to repair others and to improve and extend quality of life. Intervening in the lives of others is a challenge carrying a responsibility, again recognised long ago and addressed by Hippocrates: '*First, do no harm.*'

This starting point of care by health professionals is set out more clearly in the Hippocratic Oath (see Box 5.1). While intended for the physicians of the time, the principles encapsulated in the oath are reflective of the duties of all healthcare professionals and

---

Box 1.1 **An ancient Greek definition of happiness.**

'The good of man is the active exercise of his soul's faculties in conformity with excellence or virtue, or if there be several human excellences or virtues, in conformity with the best and most perfect among them'.

Aristotle (384–322 BCE), Nicomachean Ethics

This was paraphrased by John F. Kennedy as, 'Happiness is the full use of your powers along lines of excellence in a life affording scope'.

---

healthcare organisations in the modern era. Though modified for various settings, their essence is essentially unchanged. In the 21st century, the Physicians' Charter, a collaboration of American and European professional bodies, is a derivative of the Hippocratic Oath rather than its replacement (see Box 1.2). In addition, regulatory bodies have developed guidance on values and practice for their own disciplines which also reflect these concepts (see Further reading/resources).

Box 1.2 **The physicians' charter.**

Professionalism is the basis of medicine's contract with society.

- Fundamental principles:
  Principle of primacy of patient welfare.
  Principle of patient autonomy.
  Principle of social justice.
- A set of professional responsibilities:
  Commitment to professional competence.
  Commitment to honesty with patients.
  Commitment to patient confidentiality.
  Commitment to maintaining appropriate relations with patients.
  Commitment to improving quality of care.
  Commitment to improving access to care.

ABC of Clinical Professionalism, First Edition. Edited by Nicola Cooper, Anna Frain and John Frain.
© 2018 John Wiley & Sons Ltd. Published 2018 by John Wiley & Sons Ltd.

Commitment to a just distribution of finite resources.
Commitment to scientific knowledge.
Commitment to maintaining trust by managing conflicts of interest.
Commitment to professional responsibilities.

Adapted from ABIM Foundation, American Board of Internal Medicine, ACP-ASIM Foundation (2002) American College of Physicians-American Society of Internal Medicine, European Federation of Internal Medicine. Medical professionalism in the new millennium: A physician charter. *Annals of Internal Medicine,* **136** (3), 243–246.

Formation of professions and the duty of care

The concept of medicine as a 'profession' emerged in the late medieval period with the formation of professional guilds. Initially, the term encompassed the standards and codes of conduct of the practitioners themselves and was essentially doctor-centred. In time, the protection of medical practice from other competing professions, as well as rules governing the commercial conduct of practice, evolved the concept further. The socialisation of health services and the development of patient-centred practice in the last half-century has led to a description of professionalism as a contract between doctors and society. This contract addresses questions of funding, resource allocation and consumerism, but most importantly in ensuring that the patient's own views are heard above those of the various parties involved in healthcare. This is what Engel described as not only, '*What was the matter with the patient*', but '*what mattered to the patient*' [Engel, G.L. (1977) The need for a new medical model: a challenge for biomedicine. *Science,* **196** (4286), 129–136]. The process of healing is thus not simply the removal of disease but also the enablement of patients in achieving full use of their powers and potential (see Chapter 3).

The partnership of patient and professional has been expressed as:

Patient: I suffer; Professional: I think; Patient and Professional: We will act

(Skelton, 2002)

Even if truly patient-centred, this partnership is still potentially unequal. The patient must rely on the professional's knowledge and skills and the conscientious application of them. The patient may have insufficient expertise to adequately judge if this is the case, and so must trust his or her healthcare professional to do the right thing. In Law, this is addressed by the 'duty of care' (see Box 1.3). Both individuals and organisations control the means and manner

Box 1.3 **The duty of care.**

'Irrespective of any contract, if someone who is possessed of a special skill undertakes to apply that skill for the assistance of another person, who relies upon such skill, then a duty of care will arise'.
Lord Justice Morris, 1964
Hedley Byrne and Co. Ltd v Heller and Partners

of access to healthcare, and therefore both have a duty of care to their patients.

The employment terms and regulatory requirements for healthcare workers rest largely with providers and professional bodies. These bodies set the terms and control the application of these conditions even though professionals engage with them freely. Again, the individual trusts he/she will be dealt with fairly and his/her dignity respected. A duty of care, based on 'first, do no harm', should be firmly embedded in the culture of these organisations, for the professional remains a human being despite his/her role. Similarly, the transparency and duty of candour expected of individuals must be practiced by healthcare providers, professional bodies and other organisations which influence the delivery of healthcare.

Clinical professionalism has therefore social, ethical and legal dimensions. These dimensions serve to define society's expectations of the health professional and the constraints on the scope of clinical practice (see Chapter 9). We promote it as a positive virtue to ensure patient safety (see Chapter 7). Regulatory frameworks are also necessary to define the requirements of entry to a healthcare profession, the monitoring of continuing competence to practice and the identification of situations in which it is no longer appropriate for an individual to have professional registration (see Chapter 11). It is important to appreciate that when regulatory mechanisms are properly and compassionately applied they serve to protect not only patients but also the practitioner. This process reflects the sometime necessities of clinical practice (see Box 1.4).

Box 1.4 **Is Mr Fletcher fit to drive?**

Mr Fletcher is a 79-year-old man who lives independently with his wife. Mrs Fletcher has mobility problems due to rheumatoid arthritis and relies on her husband to drive her to social and healthcare appointments.

One evening at a traffic junction Mr Fletcher accidently goes into the back of another car. A passing Police car stops to assess the accident. There is damage to both vehicles. Mr Fletcher is noticed to be unsteady and incoherent as he gets out of the car and attempts to explain the situation. The officer breathalyses Mr Fletcher and the result is negative. However, the officer remains concerned regarding Mr Fletcher and decides to inform the Driver Vehicle Licensing Authority (DVLA). He advises Mr Fletcher to see his GP for assessment.

On seeing his GP, Mr Fletcher emphasises his need to continue driving due to his wife's needs. His wife is very vocal in her support of him. Their son is, however, concerned by his father's recent deterioration in health, and relates he has also had some problems with urinary incontinence. Mr Fletcher's GP finds him to have significant memory and concentration problems, as well as signs of Parkinson's disease. He advises Mr Fletcher he needs referral to a memory clinic and to a consultant neurologist. He tells Mr Fletcher that for the safety of himself, his wife, pedestrians and other road users, he should not drive until these assessments are complete and the DVLA has declared him fit to do so.

Although very resistant initially, Mr Fletcher and his wife conclude that his health problems do indeed make it unsafe for him to continue driving. With the support of his son, arrangements are made to provide transport for the couple when required. He surrenders his licence voluntarily. Although the insurance claim against him is on-going and stressful, on reflection he can see this situation was building for some time and perhaps he could have taken the initiative in addressing it earlier. His family and healthcare workers continue to support him in maintaining his health and quality of life as far as possible.

The agencies in this case have cooperated to ensure both Mr Fletcher's safety and that of others. A duty of care existed between each agency and Mr Fletcher to ensure he was not physically or psychologically harmed by this necessary process. These principles should inform transactions between healthcare-related organisations and individual professionals.

So what is 'clinical professionalism'?

Too often professionalism is defined by its absence. We all know when it isn't present: "*He isn't very professional*". However, having characterised the professional–patient relationship as a partnership underpinned by trust, and the professional's duty of care to the patient within a legal and regulatory framework, clinical professionalism is the mechanism by which this partnership is best guaranteed. The acquisition and application of any skill requires individual and organisational self-discipline. A common definition of medical professionalism between the various interested groups has been a work in progress. However, there is general agreement that professionalism includes:

> '*A set of values, behaviours and relationships that underpins the trust the public has in doctors*'.
> Royal College of Physicians of London, 2005

The scope of clinical professionalism has been defined by professional bodies worldwide (see Further reading/resources), but what of the public's own expectations?

The public's perspective

An online survey of 953 respondents to a 55-item inventory of professional attributes of doctors found that the public placed importance on the relationship with patients [Chandratilake, M. et al. (2010) *Clinical Medicine*, **10**, 364–369]. Doctors were expected to have high values, good behaviour and positive attitudes across personal and professional life. These roles occur in the settings of 'clinicianship', 'workmanship' and 'citizenship' (see Box 1.5). The public expects doctors to be confident, reliable, dependable, composed, accountable and dedicated across all settings. Personal appearance, physical features or social standing may play little or no role in a doctor being considered 'professional'. These attributes are exercised in varying degrees in each professional according to role, but nonetheless they overlap and interact across all settings (see Figure 1.1).

Values of workmanship and citizenship are shared with others in society and 'clinicianship' with other health professionals. Relationships and respect for fellow workers are considered

---

Box 1.5 **Public perception of medical professionalism.**

Clinicianship
- Respecting a patient's autonomy.
- Being empathic when caring for patients.
- Showing compassion towards patients.
- Being attentive to the needs of patients.
- Being accessible to patients.
- Treating patients fairly and without prejudice.
- Acting in a responsible fashion towards patients.
- Providing advice to patients and colleagues when required.
- Behaving in a reliable and dependable way.
- Communicating in a clear and effective manner.
- Showing altruism towards patients.
- Respecting patient confidentiality and privacy.
- Avoiding a cynical approach in one's job.
- Behaving with composure.

Workmanship
- Respecting colleagues.
- Treating colleagues fairly and without prejudice.
- Being attentive to the needs of colleagues.
- Working well as a member of a team.
- Acting in a responsible fashion towards colleagues.
- Treating other health professionals fairly and without prejudice.
- Being accessible to colleagues.
- Working with one's colleagues towards common goals.
- Being adaptable to changes in the workplace.
- Having the skills to train colleagues if required.
- Being able to manage situations where there is a conflict of interest.
- Having a professional attitude towards professional development.
- Showing leadership skills and initiative.
- Reflecting on one's actions with a view to improvement.
- Being receptive to constructive criticism.
- Making effective use of the resources available.
- Being aware of one's limitations as a practitioner.
- Being sensitive to the cultural background of colleagues and patients.
- Acting in a responsible fashion towards society.
- Acting with confidence in one's duties.
- Looking after one's health and well-being.
- Not using professional status for personal gain.

Citizenship
- Adhering to professional rules and regulations.
- Functioning according to the Law.
- Avoiding substance or alcohol misuse.
- Behaving honestly and with integrity.
- Being sound in judgement and in decision making.
- Taking a dedicated approach to one's work.
- Being accountable for one's actions.
- Being punctual.

Reproduced with permission from Chandratilake, M., McAleer, S., Gibson, J. and Roff, S. (2010) Medical professionalism: what does the public think? *Clinical Medicine*, **10**, 364–369.

---

important. We are both the same as other people in society but also defined particularly by our 'clinicianship', or to paraphrase Augustine of Hippo, 'With you I am a worker and citizen; for you I am a clinician'. There is both a status but also a responsibility upon the healthcare professional. While today there is necessary discussion about work–life balance which contributes to

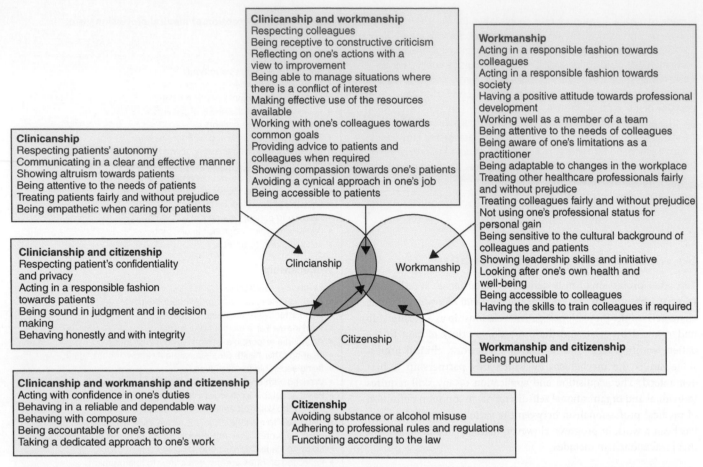

Clinicanship
Respecting patients' autonomy
Communicating in a clear and effective manner
Showing altruism towards patients
Being attentive to the needs of patients
Treating patients fairly and without prejudice
Being empathetic when caring for patients

Clinicanship and workmanship
Respecting colleagues
Being receptive to constructive criticism
Reflecting on one's actions with a view to improvement
Being able to manage situations where there is a conflict of interest
Making effective use of the resources available
Working with one's colleagues towards common goals
Providing advice to patients and colleagues when required
Showing compassion towards one's patients
Avoiding a cynical approach in one's job
Being accessible to patients

Workmanship
Acting in a responsible fashion towards colleagues
Acting in a responsible fashion towards society
Having a positive attitude towards professional development
Working well as a member of a team
Being attentive to the needs of colleagues
Being aware of one's limitations as a practitioner
Being adaptable to changes in the workplace
Treating other healthcare professionals fairly and without prejudice
Treating colleagues fairly and without prejudice
Not using one's professional status for personal gain
Being sensitive to the cultural background of colleagues and patients
Showing leadership skills and initiative
Looking after one's own health and well-being
Being accessible to colleagues
Having the skills to train colleagues if required

Clinicianship and citizenship
Respecting patient's confidentiality and privacy
Acting in a responsible fashion towards patients
Being sound in judgment and in decision making
Behaving honestly and with integrity

Clincianship

Workmanship

Citizenship

Workmanship and citizenship
Being punctual

Clinicanship and workmanship and citizenship
Acting with confidence in one's duties
Behaving in a reliable and dependable way
Behaving with composure
Being accountable for one's actions
Taking a dedicated approach to one's work

Citizenship
Avoiding substance or alcohol misuse
Adhering to professional rules and regulations
Functioning according to the law

Figure 1.1 Interaction of clinicianship, workmanship and citizenship in clinical professionalism. Reproduced with permission from Chandratilake, M., McAleer, S., Gibson, J. and Roff, S. (2010) Medical professionalism: what does the public think? *Clinical Medicine*, **10**, 364–369.

well-being, the public continues to perceive a vocational element to healthcare (from the Latin – vocare – meaning 'to call'). This is shared with other roles such as teachers and the Police. It suggests our profession is, as William Osler said, a way of life in which our role as workers, citizens and clinicians should inform our thoughts and actions in both our professional and personal lives. Indeed, our personal well-being promotes our professional well-being, and vice versa.

What of students?

Healthcare students find themselves in a position of 'proto-professionalism' – no longer members of the public but also not registered as qualified medical practitioners. They have a unique and valuable perspective on the realities of healthcare delivery, how professionalism is exercised across the three settings identified above, and their own development as professionals (see Chapter 2). Professional difficulties certainly occur during medical school, sometimes in tandem with academic and/or personal difficulty. It is important for patients, students and the profession, that students in difficulty during training are identified and supported, since issues at medical school are predictive of future performance issues [Papadakis, M.A. *et al.* (2005) Disciplinary action by medical boards and prior behaviour in medical school. *New England Journal*

of Medicine, **353**, 2673–2682]. The UK's General Medical Council has adapted its guidance '*Good Medical Practice*' for the circumstances of medical students. Professional development begins from the earliest stages of training and is context-driven. Much of this context is provided by contact with clinical teachers and doctors during training. Healthcare curricula increasingly reflect professionalism as a theme, and validated assessment tools have been developed (see Chapter 10).

Role-modelling

The acquisition of professional values is influenced significantly by a student's training environment, and particularly by the healthcare workers encountered in the early years. A role-model is often a clinical teacher (see Box 1.6). Mentioned often in the context of

Box 1.6 **Definition of role-modelling.**

'Faculty members demonstrate clinical skills, model and articulate expertise thought processes and manifest positive personal characteristics.'

From Irby, D.M. (1986) Clinical teaching and the clinical teacher. *Journal of Medical Education*, **61** (9), 35–45.

student training, role-modelling applies also post-qualification, is inter-disciplinary, occurs *by* as well as *to* the young, and between individuals and organisations.

Typically, students enter training as idealists. There may be a difference between what students are taught in formal and informal teaching and what they observe happening in practice. This is true particularly in relation to behaviours, attitudes, beliefs and values – all aspects of professionalism. Students develop their own professional behaviours from observations of their own teachers or role models. A perceived difference between what teachers say and what they do is a considerable source of student distress during training. It contributes to the perpetuation of inappropriate standards of professional behaviour among students and clinicians.

Students value any demonstration of 'altruism, responsibility, honour and integrity and respect' from their clinical teachers on the wards, and 'excellence, leadership and knowledge and skills' in the teaching/learning environment [Karnieli-Miller, O. (2011) *Academic Medicine*, **86**, 369–377]. Both, positive and negative behaviours are role-modelled by clinical teachers (see Boxes 1.7 and 1.8).

Box 1.7 Positive attributes in students' assessment of faculty professionalism.

- Takes time and effort to explain information to patients.
- Treats patients regardless of financial status, ethnic background, religious preference or sexual orientation.
- Respects patients' dignity and autonomy.
- Respects patients' confidentiality.
- Shows compassion and empathy.
- Actively listens to and shows interest in patients.
- Does not abuse power differential between teacher and student.
- Shows respectful interaction with trainees.
- Provides direction and feedback.
- Shows respectful interaction with other health professionals/other physicians.
- Admits errors or omissions.
- Shows awareness of limitations.
- Maintains appropriate boundaries.
- Avoids derogatory language.

Adapted from Todhunter, S., Cruess, S.R., Cruess, R.L. *et al.* (2011) Developing and piloting a form for student assessment of faculty professionalism. *Advances in Health Science Education*, **16**, 223–238.

Lapses of professionalism

Failing to uphold or meet the standards of behaviour expected constitutes a 'lapse'. Isolated, but significant, events arise for many reasons but require self-examination for continuing personal and professional development. They also require the support of the profession at large. Students observe lapses during their courses. They are made by fellow students, clinical teachers and administrative staff (see Figure 1.2). A consequence is an erosion of ideals and increasing cynicism about training and healthcare (see Box 1.9). This cynicism begins within the first year of training and accelerates during the first clinical (usually third) year in medicine. It falls

---

Box 1.8 Positive and negative role-modelling characteristics and behaviour identified by medical students.

Behaviour identified by students as positive (they would like to emulate in the future)	Behaviour identified by students as negative (they would not like to emulate in the future)
Clinical attributes:	
Good knowledge of general Medicine.	Inability to impart knowledge at the student level.
Articulate history taking skills.	Talking about patients without respect.
Able to explain and demonstrate clinical skills at appropriate student level.	Lack of empathy or compassion for patients.
Empathy, respect and genuine compassion for patients.	'Fake' empathy or compassion for patients
Teaching skills:	
Development of a rapport with students.	Lack of time for students within and outside of tutorials.
Provision of time towards the growth of students academically and professionally.	Poorly structured tutorials.
Provision of a positive learning environment.	Humiliation of students. Poor understanding of the curriculum and assessment requirements.
Structured tutorials with clear expectations.	Lack of meaningful feedback. Lack of patient interactions.
An understanding of the curriculum and assessment requirements.	
Immediate and meaningful feedback.	
Provision of patient interaction.	
Personal qualities:	
Respectful interdisciplinary interactions	Lack of preparation for tutorials.
Preparedness for tutorials.	Lack of enthusiasm for teaching.
Punctuality. Enthusiasm for teaching and the subject. Demonstration of a passion for their career choice.	Negative regard for other medical professionals.

Reproduced with permission from Burgess, A., Goulston, K. and Oates, K. (2015) Role modelling of clinical tutors: a focus group study among medical students. *BMC Medical Education*, **15**, 17.

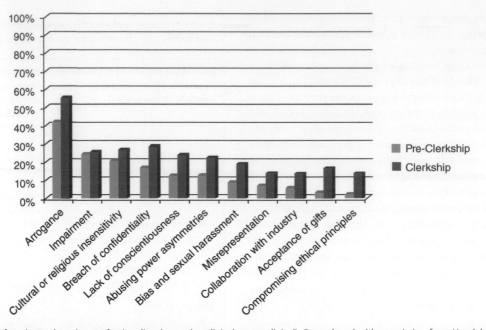

Figure 1.2 Percentage of students observing professionalism lapses (preclinical versus clinical). Reproduced with permission from Hendelman, W. and Byszewski, A. (2014) Formation of medical student professional identity: categorizing lapses of professionalism, and the learning environment. *BMC Medical Education*, **14**, 139. This is an Open Access article distributed under the terms of the Creative Commons Attribution License (http://creativecommons.org/licenses/by/4.0), which permits unrestricted use, distribution, and reproduction in any medium, provided the original work is properly credited.

Box 1.9 **Definition of cynicism.**

'A contemptuous disbelief in man's sincerity of motives or rectitude of conduct, characterized by the conviction that human conduct is suggested or directed by self-interest or self-indulgence'.

It is manifested in healthcare settings by the conduct of individuals, groups and organisations towards patients and to one another.

From Eron, L.D. (1958) The effect of medical education on attitudes: a follow up study. *Journal of Medical Education*, **33**, 25–33.

---

further in the early years of practice before rising to a more idealistic state as seniority within the profession is achieved.

The nature of lapses has altered with changing lifestyle choices and working practices. The healthcare profession was an early adopter of the internet, and there are undoubted benefits of this (see Chapter 5). In a study among United States surgical staff, 64% of junior doctors and 22% of senior doctors had Facebook pages. Of these pages, 50% were publicly accessible, and 31% of accessible pages contained work-related comments and 14% referred to specific patient situations or patient care [Landman, M. *et al.* (2010) *Journal of Surgery*, **67**, 381–386]. The high-frequency use of social networking sites may have a negative impact on medical professionalism scores, particularly integrity.

The culture of healthcare

Students begin their professional journey arguably as idealists whose professionalism is eroded by the very environment in which they aspire to work (see Chapter 6). While there are many outstanding individuals and organisations delivering exemplary patient-centred care, there is also a toxic element which damages patient care and the individuals caring for them. This toxicity encompasses many strands, but of importance are rudeness, incivility and derogatory comments, humorous or otherwise. These lapses are those which most greatly distress students. Most often derogatory comments are directed towards patients, usually out of earshot – at least of the patient – and towards fellow professionals. While most accept such comments are both disrespectful and dehumanising, at the same time they are deemed an unavoidable feature of working in a pressured environment. The airline industry is often cited as a model for risk management in healthcare. Indeed, it provides a vivid example of the effects of rudeness in healthcare (see Box 1.10).

Box 1.10 **An 'air-rage' incident.**

In 2009, two Northwest Airlines pilots flying an Airbus A320 from San Diego to Minneapolis, with 147 passengers onboard, became so engrossed in a 'heated discussion over airline policy' that they lost situational awareness and overshot the airport by 150 miles before a member of the cabin crew called the flightdeck and they realised their mistake. The flight landed safely after contact with air traffic control was resumed. The airline treated this as a serious safety incident and suspended the two pilots, whose licences were revoked. Whatever caused their lack of attention, the story illustrates the interplay between emotionally charged behaviour, namely arguing or rudeness, and cognitive skills, such as concentration.

Reproduced with permission from Flin, R. (2010) Rudeness at work. *British Medical Journal*, **340**, c2480. DOI: 10.1136/bmj.c2480.

The patient safety movement has made some impact on technological aspects of practice and systems design, but research on relational factors among staff and its impact on patient care is more limited. Among newly qualified nurses, interpersonal conflict significantly affected absenteeism, and retention of staff. Few had received training on conflict resolution or been debriefed following such incidents [McKenna, B.G., Smith, N.A., Poole, S.J. and Coverdale, J.H. (2003) Horizontal violence: experiences of registered nurses in their first year of practice. *Journal of Advanced Nursing*, **42** (1), 90–96]. The Francis Report in the UK attributed poor staff attitudes as contributory to adverse patient outcomes. A randomised controlled trial in a simulated neonatal intensive care unit examining the effect of mild rudeness on diagnostic and procedural tasks found that rudeness alone accounted for 12% of the variance between intervention and control groups. This variance increased once information sharing and seeking help were accounted for in the analysis [Riskin, A., *et al.* (2015) The impact of rudeness on medical team performance: a randomized trial. *Paediatrics*, **136** (3), 487–495].

For safe patient care, civility and respect are resources just as important as anything material or technological, and should be available in abundance. Clinical leaders should promote their positive benefits – particularly the improvement in cognitive function of healthcare staff when courtesy and consideration is practised (see Chapter 9).

Professional burnout and suicide

In 2016, *The Lancet* reported burnout among healthcare workers as having reached 'epidemic' proportions [West, C.P. *et al.* (2016) Interventions to prevent and reduce physician burnout: a systematic review and meta-analysis. *Lancet*, **388**, 2272–2281]. The evidence that those working in healthcare are being damaged by their employment is well established. It is also alarming (see Chapter 4). Despite our technological advances, it calls into question the sustainability of healthcare services, for the main method of delivery remains human to human. Suicide rates in healthcare workers are several-fold higher than in the general population, and rise further among those involved in complaints or regulatory investigations. Patients cannot be completely safe unless the safety of those treating them is also a priority.

Well-being and resilience are not simply the absence of burnout and suicidal ideas but rather 'the full use of one's powers along lines of excellence in a life affording scope' – that is, safe and successful patient care. We cannot compel resilience any more than the parents of a dysfunctional household can order their children be well-adjusted. However, we can promote it and support it both as individuals, colleagues and leaders by the manner of our conduct towards patients and professionals alike. West's systematic review of interventions to reduce burnout identifies an as-yet limited number of strategies. It is clear, however, that successful interventions are both individual-focussed as well as system and organisation-based (see Box 1.11). This implies that healthcare professionals are not the subjects of their organisations but should be working with them as equal partners. Those involved in

---

Box 1.11 **Possible strategies to prevent and reduce physician burnout.**

- Individual-focussed interventions.
  - Mindfulness
  - Stress management
- Small group discussions or curricula.
- Organisational approaches
  - Duty hour requirements
  - Locally developed modifications to clinical work processes

Adapted from West, C.P., Dyrbye, L.N., Erwin, P.J. and Shanafelt, T.D. (2016) Interventions to prevent and reduce physician burnout: a systematic review and meta-analysis. *Lancet*, **388**, 2272–2281.

---

complaints – and this means all of us at some stage – are particularly vulnerable to burnout and suicide. This should be accounted for in the structure of systems and organisations (see Further reading/resources). While responsibility must be assumed where responsibility lies, exclusive focus on the perceived shortcomings of an individual produces personal and professional isolation for that person with sometimes devastating consequences for the individuals, their family and friends. Attention focussed solely on individuals can overlook the systematic or organisational issues contributing to clinical error, and thus make its repetition more likely [Reason, J. (2000) Human error: models and management. *British Medical Journal*, **320**, 768–770].

Conclusions

The clinician–patient relationship remains the keystone of healthcare delivery. A duty of care occurs at each interaction with patients, but arises also in how professionals relate to one another and how healthcare organisations relate to those delivering services to patients. Civility and respect are fundamental principles of clinical professionalism and essential to increasing patient safety. The alternative is cynicism and burnout, which potentially damages everyone. Clinical leaders should be person-centred and motivated to bring about the full use of professionals' powers along lines of excellence in the best interests of patient care.

Further reading/resources

ABIM Foundation, American Board of Internal Medicine, ACP-ASIM Foundation (2002) American College of Physicians-American Society of Internal Medicine, European Federation of Internal Medicine. Medical professionalism in the new millennium: A physician charter. *Annals of Internal Medicine*, **136** (3), 243–246.

Chandratilake, M., McAleer, S., Gibson, J. and Roff, S. (2010) Medical professionalism: what does the public think? *Clinical Medicine*, **10**, 364–369.

Papadakis, M.A., Teherani, A., Banach, M.A. *et al.* (2005) Disciplinary action by medical boards and prior behaviour in medical school. *New England Journal of Medicine*, **353**, 2673–2682.

Karnieli-Miller, O., Vu, R., Frankel, R.M. *et al.* (2011) Which experiences in the hidden curriculum teach students about professionalism? *Academic Medicine*, **86**, 369–377.

Landman, M., Shelton, J., Kauffmann, R.M. (2010) Guidelines for maintaining a professional compass in the era of social networking. *Journal of Surgery*, **67**, 381–386.

Riskin, A., Erez, A., Foulk, T.A. *et al.* (2015) The impact of rudeness on medical team performance: a randomised trial. *Pediatrics*, **136** (3), 487–495.

West, C.P., Dyrbye, L.N., Erwin, P.J. and Shanafelt, T.D. (2016) Interventions to prevent and reduce physician burnout: a systematic review and meta-analysis. *Lancet*, **388**, 2272–2281.

CHAPTER 2

Acquiring and Developing Professional Values

Sue Murphy[1], Alison Greig[1] and Anna Frain[2]

[1] Department of Physical Therapy, University of British Columbia, Canada
[2] Division of Health Sciences and Graduate Entry Medicine, University of Nottingham, UK

OVERVIEW

- Professionalism is accepted as a core value for clinical professionals and needs to be taught in health professional programmes.
- The concepts of apprenticeship, role-modelling and the hidden curriculum are explored in the context of the teaching of professionalism.
- Workload and systemic issues can be barriers to the development of professionalism.
- Reflection and interprofessional learning are valuable elements of teaching and developing professionalism.
- Self-care is an often forgotten but essential part of acquiring and developing professional values.

Box 2.1 The American Physical Therapy Association (APTA) core values on professionalism.

1 Accountability.
2 Altruism.
3 Compassion/caring.
4 Excellence.
5 Integrity.
6 Professional duty.
7 Social responsibility.

Adapted from Professionalism in Physical Therapies: Core Values (pdf), http://www.apta.org/Professionalism/. Accessed on 22 April 2017.

Introduction

The values of any health professional are grounded in a commitment of care for others, and underpin the trust the public has in healthcare providers. Across the health professions, there are shared generic values, which often include altruism, excellence, accountability, integrity, professional duty and social responsibility (see Box 2.1). While values are learned and arise from personal experience, there is a need to foster the development of professional values in healthcare providers throughout their careers. Programmes can begin to identify desired values through an appropriate selection of students, and then further foster and assess the ongoing development of desired values through educational practices. Professional values are integral to the formation of professional identity, and are fundamental to decision-making in clinical practice.

Professionalism as a competency

Professionalism and professional behaviour may be seen as competencies that can be learned and demonstrated. Miller's Pyramid (see Figure 2.1) can be used to illustrate the progression of competency, with 'does' representing the highest level of performance.

Despite many health professions having 'professionalism' as a core requirement of entry-level practice, there is little consensus on optimal teaching strategies to develop competence in professionalism. This is further explored in Chapter 10. However, it is well recognised that socialisation in clinical and professional settings plays a key role in the development of professional behaviours such as communication, collaboration, respect, teamwork, and the ability to maintain professional boundaries.

Students who do not develop competence in professional behaviours during training may struggle with professionalism in their early careers, where mentorship may focus more on the development of technical skills, as opposed to fostering professional qualities (see Figure 2.2).

ABC of Clinical Professionalism, First Edition. Edited by Nicola Cooper, Anna Frain and John Frain.
© 2018 John Wiley & Sons Ltd. Published 2018 by John Wiley & Sons Ltd.

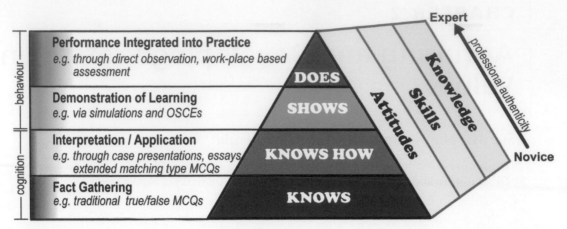

Figure 2.1 Miller's Prism of Clinical Competence (it is only in the 'does' triangle that true performance occurs). Reproduced with kind permission from Mehay R and Burns R. (2009). Assessment and competence. In Mehay R [Ed]: The Essential Handbook for GP Training and Education. Also available at: http://www. essentialgptrainingbook.com/chapter-29.php. (Accessed August 2017).

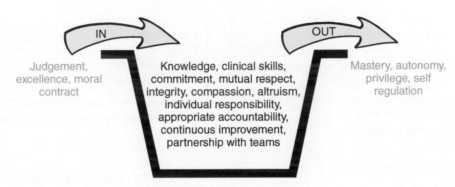

Figure 2.2 The basket of professional qualities. Reproduced with permission from Wass, V. (2006) Doctors in society: medical professionalism in a changing world. *Clinical Medicine*, **6** (1), 109–113.

The development of professional identity

The development of professional identity begins on admission to professional training and continues throughout a clinician's professional life. The personal values that the practitioner brings to their professional lives contribute to professional identity. However, the development of an individual's professional identity – or who they are in their professional role – is complex.

The experiences of an individual health professional, including interactions with patients and professional communities of practice, and the transition from student to practising clinician, can be integral to identity development. Critical incidents in the clinical setting may also influence identity formation during the career pathway.

Some authors (see Further reading/resources) have argued that professional identity is the final level of achievement of professional competence; however, others believe that professional identity formation is a distinct developmental process which must be encouraged and supported throughout a professional's training and career.

The traditional apprenticeship

Although the term 'traditional apprenticeship' might conjure up images of a skilled tradesman mentoring a junior worker, the supervised clinical practice of those entering the health professions is essentially a traditional apprenticeship. An apprenticeship involves a novice learning from an expert in the context in which they will eventually become an expert themselves. The skills learned during an apprenticeship are not only technical (i.e., clinical skills). Attitudes, behaviours, language and values – including professional values – are learned through the formal and informal observation of others, through demonstration, and through the assignment of tasks with increasing autonomy and complexity. For an apprenticeship to be successful, novices need to spend a significant period of time with one or two mentors, rather than spend short blocks of time with several different teachers.

Role models

Expert professionals often act as role models for other members of the healthcare team, including students. Observation of the professional behaviour of others with patients, and in the

Box 2.2 **Case history: Appropriate behaviour in one context may be inappropriate in another, and difficult to distinguish for novices.**

Patient Will Smith has been seeing Dr Jones for many years for a chronic condition. Over the years Dr Jones has got to know Will and his family well. Dr Jones started her interaction with Will by asking about his daughter's progress at school, and whether his golf had improved. Jonas Blake, a medical student observing the interaction, saw that these personal questions built rapport with Will, and imitated this approach in his next encounter with a new patient. Jonas was horrified when the new patient lodged a complaint, saying that the student was unprofessional and asked irrelevant personal questions.

Box 2.3 **The impact of the hidden curriculum versus the formal curriculum.**

Case history: Breach of confidentiality.

Jonathan Blake was on his first day of a clinical rotation as a physiotherapy student. He had reviewed the orientation materials he was provided with, including the rules on confidentiality. He remembered how important it was never to divulge any details about patients in public under any circumstances.

As he travelled in the lift to start his shift on the first morning, he heard several staff discussing patients by name, while standing next to a notice reminding people about confidentiality. Although he was initially concerned about this apparent breach of professional behaviour, after several days of repeated experiences he found himself doing the same thing.

clinical context in general, provides a powerful influence, particularly if that professional is seen as a role model. Role models can portray positive or negative professional behaviour, either of which may be emulated by other team members. Reasons for the significant impact of role models vary, but may include a desire to 'fit in' with the rest of the team, to obtain perceived status or approval from a superior, or because it is simply 'the way people behave around here'. Some less-experienced clinicians may imitate the professional behaviour of role models and inappropriately transpose it to a new setting because of their lack of understanding of the contextual factors which influence practice in a specific situation. Transposing observed practice to a different context may turn actions from being appropriate to inappropriate (see Box 2.2).

When clinicians or mentors realise they have demonstrated breaches in professional behaviour, positive role-modelling can still occur by open discussion of how the situation could have been handled differently, and what some of the causal factors of the inappropriate behaviour might have been. This role models reflective practice, lifelong learning and continual self-improvement.

The hidden curriculum

As role models, expert clinicians and teachers do not always appreciate that students learn by their example even when they are not formally teaching. This area of unintended learning in the clinical or educational environment is known as the 'hidden curriculum'.

Learners may perceive this learning as more credible than formal learning, and it may be a powerful influence on behaviour. In the clinical setting the hidden curriculum provides clues and cues as to acceptable or preferred standards of professional behaviour which may be contradictory to what is learned in an academic environment, or what is stated in professional standards or regulations. Many students are taught about professionalism in the early phases of their education; they later move into the clinical world and find what they see does not match up with what they have learned (see Box 2.3).

Within the clinical world, factors such as time pressure, excessive workload, administrative requirements and other system pressures

contribute to the hidden curriculum and can create an environment in which adhering to espoused professional values can be challenging – and in extreme cases rewards violation of those values. Honest and open discussion of the hidden curriculum in a clinical context can help clinicians become aware of what they are learning, and what effect this is having on their professional values. If not addressed overtly, the hidden curriculum may communicate that professionalism is not important, leading to poor professional behaviour which may go unchallenged.

Barriers to developing professional values

Apprenticeships, role models and the hidden curriculum contribute to what Coulehan (see Further reading/resources), who has a background in the humanities, calls 'narrative-based professionalism', in contrast to 'rule-based professionalism'. 'Rule-based professionalism' describes a set of objectives, competencies and measurable behaviours that attempt to capture the concept of professionalism, but which may not focus on what it really means. By using 'narrative-based professionalism' such as stories or case histories students can discuss and reflect on areas which are not totally black and white. They can test their understanding in a deeper and more practical way in areas of professionalism which are less easily measured.

In terms of medical education there is clear evidence that professionalism reduces during medical school. This can be demonstrated as early as the first year of study in both the USA and United Kingdom [Humprey, H.J. *et al.* (2007) Promoting an environment of professionalism: the University of Chicago "roadmap". *Academic Medicine*, **82** (11), 1098–1107; Frain, A., unpublished data). Some examples have been given in Boxes 2.4 and 2.5 of case histories where role modelling, the professionalism gap and the hidden curriculum have both positive and negative influences.

In Box 2.6, evidence is being gathered about how current medical students' understanding and experience of professionalism has been developing throughout their course.

Box 2.4 **The professionalism gap experienced by students.**

Case history: Poor professionalism and infection control.

Andy was on his first clinical placement in his physiotherapy programme. He was excited and nervous to be actually seeing patients. His first professionalism session was called, 'First do no harm', and emphasised the importance of infection control when seeing patients. Andy washed his hands before and after seeing each patient. However, he felt very uncomfortable that the physiotherapist he was shadowing did not wash his hands more than twice in the whole morning. Shouldn't he say something? Gradually he began to feel embarrassed and washed his hands less and less. By the end of the session he felt confused and disappointed. He felt he had not learnt anything because he was so preoccupied about hand washing.

Case history: Poor communication and lack of empathy.

Gemma, a third year student nurse, was scrubbed up in theatre assisting a surgeon as part of her clinical attachment in vascular surgery. She was shocked and distressed at the way the patient was spoken to by the surgeon on the ward round earlier that day. She detected a lack of empathy and felt that the patient was ill at ease. She wanted to talk with the surgeon about it but felt unable to do so because she perceived him to be very senior and unapproachable.

Box 2.5 **The influence of role models on choice of speciality.**

Case history: An inspirational role model.

During a workshop for final-year nursing students, there was a discussion of choice of preferred clinical speciality. Everyone was surprised when Ed said he wanted to work in palliative care. One of his colleagues thought it would be too depressing and difficult, and wondered why Ed was so certain. They were moved when he told them about the MacMillan Nurse Temi on his first placement two-and-a-half years ago. Even after all this time, Ed remained inspired by the care and kindness as well as the skills and knowledge demonstrated by Temi during those 8 weeks.

Case history: How not to inspire the next generation of GPs.

Alice is a General Practitioner and a clinical skills tutor. She expresses her frustration to some of the medical students about the minutiae of rules and regulations that a GP needs to adhere to these days. One particular problem was a health and safety policy ensuring that staff did not walk and talk at the same time if carrying equipment, and another which was a 'ladder policy'.

Three years later, Alice bumps into a student who is approaching finals and asks about his career choice. He wants to go into hospital medicine. She asks if he has considered being a GP. He quotes back their conversation three years previously, and says ever since that day he has thought being a GP was just too frustrating and full of unnecessary policies. Alice feels very guilty that her thoughtless words have had such an impact.

Box 2.6 **Evidence of how professionalism values develop during graduate entry medical school.**

A qualitative study is ongoing in a UK medical school interviewing eight graduate entry medical students throughout their training. Themes have emerged reflecting differing attitudes to and understanding of professionalism as the course progresses.

Influences from previous careers are apparent in their early understanding of professionalism. They pick up understanding of specific areas of professionalism such as confidentiality and use of social media from teaching during the first 18 months of the course. The students start to realise that even seemingly obvious things such a private face-book setting is essential, and that patient-identifiable paperwork, conversations and social media postings are unacceptable.

As they move into the clinical course, role-modelling and the hidden curriculum are foremost in their interviews. They move from idealists to pragmatists, understanding human factors in themselves and professionals and colleagues with whom they are working. They recount many examples of both good professionalism as well as lapses by themselves, colleagues and teachers/clinicians they have experienced during their course.

Further analysis is taking place on the interview material, but so far the results seem to suggest an increased understanding of rather than a decline in professionalism of the students during their medical school career.

Reflection and professional development

The importance of reflection and reflective practice, including reflection on aspects of practice related to professionalism (e.g., communication, advocacy and conflict resolution) is an important part of lifelong learning and the development of professional competencies and professional identity. Educators assert that reflective practice encourages students to act and to think professionally, and is an integral part of health professional education. The development of professional identity requires understanding one's personal beliefs, attitudes and values in the context of the professional culture. Reflection offers an explicit approach to developing this understanding.

Novices typically reflect 'on' action, and need time to reflect on professional interactions *after* they occur to determine any possible pros and cons of the action taken, and to develop alternative courses of more favourable action for next time. More experienced clinicians may be able to reflect 'in' action, and are hence able to adjust their behaviour and approach *during* a clinical encounter. Reflection requires time, which is often lacking in clinical settings, and is often most valuable when it is a guided process with a mentor or colleague who can probe, clarify, or push for more depth or an alternate perspective on an issue. Although reflection on clinical encounters is relatively common, the focus is often on technical (clinical) skills rather than professional aspects of the encounter such as communication, respect for the patient, and understanding cultural diversity. A lack of focus and reflection on these aspects can make professionalism and professional values appear

Box 2.7 **Case-Based Discussion (CBD): An example of integrating reflection on technical skills and professionalism in the same case.**

Jenny, a third-year nursing student has to choose a particular patient she has seen in the last week of her attachment. Her mentor asks her to look at one which was challenging from different aspects, not only in the skills Jenny had demonstrated in communication and examination as well as knowledge of the condition, but also professionalism issues. Jenny chose the following case.

- Mrs B came to see the practice nurse for her dressings. Mrs B arrived late. She had missed her last two appointments and was quite abusive to Jenny and the practice nurse. There were some very dirty dressings on her legs which were almost falling off. Mrs B's son, who was a drug addict, accompanied her and demanded to have some information about his partner while he was in the consultation. It happened that Jenny had seen his partner the previous day.
- The dressings were complex and Mrs B's legs were red and swollen. She seemed confused and unwell.

Jenny's mentor was able to address the following issues with her:

1 The information gathered from Jenny and recorded in the notes.
2 The examination, including observations of the legs but also vital signs.
3 Jenny's understanding of asking for help from a more senior clinician as the patient was unwell.
4 How to cope with a patient who arrives late.
5 How to manage a non-complaint patient.
6 Confidentiality issues around the son's demands.
7 Her attitude and feelings when the patient was aggressive – how did she handle this?
8 How to manage a vulnerable patient.

In this way, Jenny can use the CBD to reflect on technical and professional skills she is acquiring.

Box 2.8 **Canadian Inter-Professional Health Collaborative's six domains of competency.**

Effective inter-professional working requires good:

1 Clarification of roles.
2 Team functioning.
3 Patient/client/family/community centredness.
4 Collaborative leadership.
5 Inter-professional communication.
6 Inter-professional conflict resolution.

Adapted from www.cihc.ca. Accessed 22 April 2017.

- Improved patient safety and communication among healthcare providers.
- More efficient and effective employment of health human resources.
- Improved satisfaction among patients and healthcare providers.

According to the Canadian Interprofessional Health Collaborative, inter-professional collaboration requires competency in six domains, illustrated in Box 2.8.

Effective inter-professional collaboration requires shared values, interdependence, constructive handling of differences, joint ownership of decisions and collective responsibility for outcomes. A core set of shared values for professionalism can provide a framework through which students and clinicians can form respectful relationships with both patients and other healthcare professionals. Breakdowns in inter-professional collaboration and team functioning can occur when there is abuse of power, arrogance, misrepresentation, lack of conscientiousness and conflicts of interest. These personal, value-based factors emphasise the need for healthcare professionals to be reflective and aware of their own behaviour and its impact on others.

Self-care in the maintenance of professionalism

Workload, financial pressures, targets and under resourcing result in a culture that implies a set of values that diametrically oppose those taught as core to professionalism. Novice health professionals may experience internal conflict as they try to reconcile the explicit and hidden curricula. Self-care is an essential but often forgotten aspect of professionalism, which impacts resilience, or the capacity to deal with difficulties, and is vital in a profession whose core values include altruism and compassion (see Box 2.9).

Box 2.9 **Case history: The importance of self-care.**

Fiona is an experienced Advanced Nurse Practitioner. She started to get recurrent urinary infections which required repeated antibiotics. She noticed there was a clear pattern – her 12 hour shifts running the Emergency Clinic always resulted in frequency and dysuria. She knew she must drink more, and go to pass urine as soon as she needed to, but somehow she could not manage to do this. In the end she required long-term sick leave because of significant renal problems, resulting in great distress to her and staffing issues in the clinic.

secondary to the 'real' point of the clinical encounter. Focussed reflection on professional aspects of an encounter can help to provide insights into how they might be improved or varied in different clinical situations. An example of such a focussed reflection, combining both technical skills and professionalism in the same case reflection, is shown in Box 2.7.

Inter-professional collaboration and professionalism

Many of the attributes that health professionals develop relate to values, professional competence and professional identity highlighted during interactions with the inter-professional team.

The benefits of effective inter-professional collaboration and teamwork are well supported in the literature, and include the following:

- Improved population healthcare/patient care.
- Improved access to healthcare.
- Improved recruitment and retention of healthcare providers.

That fact that clinical care can have a profound effect on the physical and mental health of a professional, and hence on empathy and professionalism, has been long recognised:

> 'My wife and I had to come to realize one of the chief difficulties of the family doctor – the constant drain upon the emotions. To stand helplessly while relentless organisms destroy a beautiful mother, a fine father, or a beloved child, creates terrible emotional distress; and this feeling is increased by the necessity of suppression. That is why the average lifetime of family doctors is 55 years, most of them succumbing to functional impairment.'
>
> Joseph Jerger, MD, written in 1939. http://doctorspage.net/satisf.asp (accessed 25 April 2017).

Ballatt and Campling (see Further reading/resources) suggest that, 'Kindness to patients will be more sustainable if staff are self-aware and able to treat themselves more kindly'. There is ample evidence in the public inquiry in to the Mid Staffordshire NHS Foundation Trust (see Further reading/resources) which indicates that failure of self-care can lead to an erosion of empathy and eventually burnout (a topic that is explored further in Chapter 4). This can result in unprofessional behaviour and have a disastrous effect on patient care.

Building an awareness of the importance of self-care during training is important. The Royal Australian College of General Practitioners recognises that health professionals cannot give to others if they are experiencing 'compassion fatigue', and has advised that self-care and a 'whole of practice approach' be addressed so that patients receive the best care. It describes self-care as an essential element of professional life.

Lotte Dyrbye suggests a 'two-bucket approach' to promote wellbeing which is summarised in Boxes 2.10 and 2.11.

In his book, *When Breath Becomes Air*, the neurosurgeon Paul Kalanathi acknowledges the dilemma of choosing one's medical

---

Box 2.10 Bucket No 1: Taking personal responsibility for self-care, happiness.

Set time each week to pursue a duty at your practice that you enjoy	We generally have something at work we enjoy most – it could be patient care, an aspect of administration or striving for improvements. Finding meaning in our work makes us more satisfied and less likely to become cynical.
Actually take holidays	Back in the 1990s consultants encouraged juniors to work during their holidays, and it is surprising how many clinicians still do not take all their holidays. We prioritise work over personal satisfaction.
Maintain a healthy diet and exercise	There is evidence that if we practice what we preach to our patients we are less likely to experience burnout.
Talk to your spouse	Communication can help minimise work–home conflicts, one of the key drivers of burnout.
Avoid delayed gratification	Many professionals will recognise the fact that we put off hobbies and leisure activities and put work first repeatedly. We will be better able to care for our patients if we have a good balance and should not wait until we retire to do these things.

Reproduced with permission from Dyrbye, L. 2015. Two-bucket approach to promote wellbeing. https://wire.ama-assn.org/ama-news/burnout-busters-how-boost-satisfaction-personal-life-practice. Accessed 25 April 2017.

Box 2.11 Bucket No 2: Establishing an environment of wellness.

Offer honest discussions	Within an organisation, recognising the need for self-care and avoiding each member of a team trying to work this out in isolation can improve the function of the team and improve patient care.
Encourage physicians to talk about medical errors	We know that when doctors talk about medical errors, it can help prevent future errors and reduce inappropriate self-blame and distress.
Build a wellness index or tool to help physicians properly assess their risks for burnout	Despite having the ability to assess patients' needs, physicians often struggle to assess their own well-being and stress. Dyrbye quotes the use of a wellness index amongst surgeons* and suggests we consider using a tool for self assessment.
Develop flexible schedules	In hospitals and practices that are able, flexible work schedules and systems that facilitate hand-offs can alleviate the 'exorbitant responsibility to work all hours'.

*In a 2013 study of 1150 participants, the surgeons' personal assessment of well-being relative to colleagues was poor. Among the participants, 89% of surgeons believed their well-being was at or above average, including 70.5% with scores in the bottom 30% relative to national norms. After receiving objective, individualised feedback based on the Mayo Clinic Physician Well-Being Index score, 46.6% of these surgeons indicated that they intended to make specific life changes. Source: Shanafelt, T.D., Kaups, K.L., Nelson, H. *et al.* An Interactive Individualized Intervention to Promote Behavioral Change to Increase Personal Well-Being in US Surgeons. *Annals of Surgery* 2014;**259** (1):82–88.

Reproduced with permission from Dyrbye, L. (2015) Two-bucket approach to promote wellbeing. https://wire.ama-assn.org/ama-news/burnout-busters-how-boost-satisfaction-personal-life-practice. Accessed 25 April 2017.

speciality. He writes: 'Putting lifestyle first is how you find a job – not a calling'. It is intangibly recognised that being a member of a healthcare profession is more than just a job, and yet the modern healthcare environment requires balance in order to be able to maintain resilience and professionalism (see Box 2.12).

Box 2.12 **Balance is the key.**

Case history: Burn out in a clinician.

Phil, an experienced Advanced Nurse Practitioner, loved his job and was very good at it. He noticed he was losing weight and having trouble sleeping. He felt the weekends were not long enough, and he did not feel refreshed by the time Monday morning came along. He was shocked when a complaint arrived from a colleague about the way he handled a patient with rectal bleeding. The patient did not come to harm, but the colleague was worried that Phil did not follow guidelines.

The team had a meeting where they discussed the situation. They were very supportive and understanding. What emerged was that Phil has been trying to shoulder the burden of the difficulties the practice had been experiencing with recruitment by working extra-long days and not taking holidays (he was due 6 weeks a year and took only 3 weeks). An audit revealed that Phil had seen the most patients, worked the longest hours, and taken the least holidays. Kath, another Advanced Nurse Practitioner, had seen the least patients, taken all the holidays she was entitled to ensuring all her next years' holidays were also booked and agreed, and worked the least hours.

The error was discussed and the team resolved that Phil would try to improve his self-care, including taking all of his holidays. Kath agreed to share the additional workload and encourage Phil to be as proactive as her in regards to holidays and protecting himself from excess stress. The practice took their share of the responsibility for the situation, and a robust recruitment strategy was developed.

Conclusions

Professionalism can be seen as seen as a set of competencies that can be learned and demonstrated; however, the development of professional identity goes beyond that. Values internal to the goals of the profession and a commitment to moral behaviour grounded in 'that which I hold most sacred' (to quote a contemporary version of the Hippocratic Oath), as well as a sharing of these values and beliefs, leads to a strong sense of professional community identity. Values, beliefs and community are essential components of healthcare professionalism. However modern healthcare, with all its pressures, opposes professionalism in many ways. A focus on professionalism, including role-modelling, recognition and management of the hidden curriculum, narrative competence, reflection on professional issues and self-care, are increasingly important in the acquisition, development and maintenance of professional values.

Further reading/resources

Cruess, R.L., Cruess, S.R. and Steinert, Y. (2016) Amending Miller's Pyramid to include professional identity formation. *Academic Medicine*, **91** (2), 180–185.

Coulehan, J. (2005) Viewpoint: today's professionalism: engaging the mind but not the heart. *Academic Medicine*, **80** (10), 892–898.

Ballatt, J. and Campling, P. (2011) *Intelligent Kindness. Reforming the culture of healthcare*. RCPsych Publications, London.

Kalanithi, P. (2016) *When Breath Becomes Air*. The Bodley Head, London.

The Canadian Interprofessional Health Collaborative. Available at: www.cihc. ca (accessed December 2016).

The Mid Staffordshire NHS Foundation Trust Public Enquiry, chaired by Robert Francis QC. Department of Health, 2013. http://webarchive.nationalarchives. gov.uk/20150407084003/http://www.midstaffspublicinquiry.com (accessed December 2016).

CHAPTER 3

Patient-Centred Care

Anna Frain[1] and Andy Wearn[2]

[1] Division of Medical Sciences and Graduate Entry Medicine, University of Nottingham, UK
[2] Clinical Skills Centre, Faculty of Medicine and Health Sciences, The University of Auckland, New Zealand

---

OVERVIEW

- Traditional, 'paternalistic' clinician-centred care is moving towards patient-centred care in many countries.
- The fundamental starting point of patient-centred care is respect for the patient as a person.
- Good communication, including listening skills, use of appropriate language and empathy, is essential.
- Consent and capacity must be addressed as well as practising shared decision-making with patients.
- Reflection and values-based practice are helpful ways of learning and practising patient-centred care.
- Practising patient-centred care is particularly important for those who are vulnerable (e.g., due to age, language or capacity).

Clinician-centred care

'The good physician treats the disease. The great physician treats the patient who has the disease.'

'It is much more important to know what sort of a patient has a disease than what sort of a disease a patient has.'

Sir William Osler, physician (1849–1919)

Historically, clinical professionals have been regarded as highly trained and skilled, attracting respect and admiration from their patients. A consequence of this was a reluctance to question their advice and decisions. This style of care has been described as 'beneficent paternalism' – acting on behalf of or for the good of patients.

In practice, some patients feel more confident in a clinician who advises what to do and what is 'best for them'. Making a decision about treatment can be stressful for the patient, but may also reflect poor preparation and explanation by the professional involved, with a lack of commitment and time given to this process. This state of affairs can be perpetuated by clinician style. A 1996 study showed that oncologists using closed questions made it more difficult for patients to start any discussion. Only 1% of questions were related to patient concerns, and the frequency of expressed empathy from the doctors in this study was as low as 1%.

This type of clinician-centred care is no longer acceptable or desirable in many countries, and there has been a move to a more patient-centred paradigm of healthcare. This shift has probably been driven by broader societal change as well as a reframing of professional practice from a focus on the features of the profession to the acts of the professional.

The evolution of patient-centred care

Dr Paul Kalanathi, in his book, *When Breath Becomes Air* (see Further reading/resources), gives the early definition of 'patient' as 'one who endures hardship without complaint' or being 'the object of an action' – from the Latin word *patio* (I suffer) – which is how he felt as his own cancer progressed.

Taking this context of serious illness as an example, a 2005 study found that 98% of patients wanted their doctor to be realistic when breaking bad news. In a 2001 study of 2231 cancer patients, 87% wanted as much information as possible – good or bad – and 98% wanted to know if they had 'cancer'. If we listen to our patients and have them at the centre of our care we will be better able to respond appropriately (see Box 3.1).

Box 3.1 Inspirational patient-centred care.

Dr Paul Kalanathi was inspired to become a neurosurgeon in part by watching a paediatric neurosurgeon talking with the parents of a child with a brain tumour. *'He not only delivered the clinical facts but addressed the human facts as well, acknowledging the tragedy of the situation and providing guidance'.* The patient and family were at the centre of his care.

Kalanathi, P. (2016) *When Breath Becomes Air.* Bodley Head, London.

ABC of Clinical Professionalism, First Edition. Edited by Nicola Cooper, Anna Frain and John Frain.
© 2018 John Wiley & Sons Ltd. Published 2018 by John Wiley & Sons Ltd.

Developments in patient-centred care reflect changes in society as well as expectations of patients and clinicians. However, patients being at the centre of care must not just be a theoretical promise but an actual change in attitude.

In 2002, Skelton *et al.* summarised the archetypal doctor patient interjection as: 'I (patient) suffer, I (doctor) think, we will act'. It is helpful to reflect on our own experiences as clinicians and students, about the way we ourselves and others treat patients. Is the care we give and witness truly patient-centred (see Box 3.2)?

Communication skills

Good communications skills are essential for patient-centred care. Combining biomedical and psychosocial models of communications enables us not only to discover what is the matter with the patient, but also, as Engel described, 'what matters *to* the patient'.

Remembering to reflect on the consultation as an interaction between two human beings allows us to communicate on a level playing field – what Berne described as a functional adult-to-adult interaction.

Listening

> '*Listen to the patient; he is telling you the diagnosis*'.
> Sir William Osler

Studies show that 70–90% of diagnoses are made on the history alone. This is as true today as when it was first reported in 1975, even with advances in technology. There are many distractions that

reduce our attention, including computers, interruptions, targets, and simply the awareness of how many patients are waiting to be seen. Yet, if we *listen*, our examination, investigations and differential diagnoses will be more targeted and accurate. The 'golden minute' of just listening at the start of a consultation actually speeds up the consultation, allowing the patient's agenda to be revealed. When clinicians are in a hurry, they listen less and consultations take longer (see Box 3.3).

Empathy

Empathy is, according to the *Oxford English Dictionary*, 'the power of identifying oneself with, and so fully comprehending, the person who is the subject of contemplation'.

Author Paul Kalanithi was surprised that, after years of working as a doctor, it was only as a patient that he discovered simple things such as how painful and difficult physiotherapy can be. We may not be able to directly put ourselves in our patients' shoes, but we can draw on our own experiences and we can ask about theirs (see Box 3.4).

For most people, empathy is a natural emotion, but for others it is more difficult and requires nurturing. As with all communication skills, clinicians can learn to incorporate empathy meaningfully in their practice.

However, the reality is that clinical practice can erode empathy – one sign of burnout is a loss of empathy (see Chapter 4). When we are exhausted and overstretched, empathy is a casualty, so self-care and self-awareness are important in maintaining this key aspect of patient-centred care.

Retaining a degree of professional detachment is also important. In a teaching video about dying of cancer, a patient who was also a nurse explained that the relationship she had with professionals caring for her was totally different to that of her friends and family, and the separation was clear. Understanding and respecting this is an important lesson for all clinicians. We may feel emotions such as sadness, distress or anger about particular patients, and this is normal. There is a 'dance' that we participate in, between appropriate empathy and over-involvement, and we take each step with care.

Using everyday language

Students in the health professions learn a new language from the start of their course. It is surprising how quickly we forget everyday language and use jargon. Terms such as benign, malignant, bacteria or virus may be difficult to navigate even for a highly intelligent patient. Names of drugs can be unpronounceable or very similar. Patients may be too nervous to ask us to clarify what we mean.

Patient-centred care requires us to check our patients' understanding. Patients retain only a small percentage of what is discussed in a consultation, and if jargon is used even less will be remembered and acted upon. Clinicians often underestimate the intelligence of their patients, but may overestimate their understanding of medical terminology. For example, we forget that a 'scan' could mean a dozen different tests, and if we do not clarify what we mean patients may make uninformed decisions or face a surprise. In some ways health professionals act as an interpreter, ensuring that jargon is explained and the patient has understood what is being said.

Consent to examination and treatment

In patient-centred care the knowledge of the clinician and the needs and wishes of the patient combine. Consent is an area in which clinical, cultural, ethical, moral and legal matters overlap (discussed further in Chapter 9). Respect for the patient and their rights lies at the centre of this issue. All the relevant information should be provided in an easy-to-understand and accessible format. Informing patients and involving them in decisions is integral to their care (see Box 3.5).

Box 3.5 Failure to gain valid consent by not checking a patient's understanding.

Mrs Summers was seen by a nurse and advised that a ring pessary might help her vaginal prolapse. When she came to see the general practitioner there was no information in the patient notes, and Mrs Summers simply dangled the pessary in front of the doctor.

The doctor was busy and not expecting a procedure. He was also unclear as to what the problem was, who had suggested the procedure, and why the patient had not been booked with a chaperone. Mrs Summers was not clear what she was going to have done.

The doctor realised Mrs Summers was anxious and uncertain about what the procedure would involve, so he decided not to go ahead in order to discuss properly what it would involve, gain informed consent, and re-book the procedure with a chaperone.

Box 3.6 Principles of the Mental Capacity Act (England & Wales 2005).

The Mental Capacity Act was introduced to protect vulnerable adults. The Act authorises a clinician to act or treat, as long as the principles of the Mental Capacity Act are observed, 'reasonable steps' have been made to ascertain decision-making capacity, and the assessment has led to a 'reasonable belief' that the person lacks capacity in relation to the matter in question.

The Act is underpinned by five principles:

- Presumption of capacity.
- Support in decision-making.
- Acceptance of unwise decisions.
- Acting in best interests.
- Taking the least restrictive option.

Consent can be implied, for example, when a patient puts out their arm for a nurse to check their blood pressure. It can be verbal, for example, when a patient agrees to have a cervical smear test (but this should be documented in the patient's notes, including the offer of a chaperone). Written consent is required for invasive procedures, for example gastroscopy or surgery, or enrolment in a clinical trial. Ideally, the clinician recommending or carrying out the treatment should be the one to gain consent, although this can be delegated to other competent clinicians. However, it is important to understand that patients (other than, for example, those detained under the Mental Health Act in England) have the right to refuse all or part of information and treatment. If this is the case, it should be documented.

For consent to be valid, it should not only be informed but the patient should also have the mental capacity to understand, retain and weigh up the information in order to make a decision. Different countries have different legal frameworks regarding mental capacity. In England, any person over the age of 16 years is assumed to have capacity unless, on the balance of probabilities, they are judged not to (see Box 3.6).

Unexpected or irrational decisions do not necessarily mean a patient lacks capacity, but it might indicate that further explanation and understanding is required. Values-based practice means we should try to understand the patient's perspective and not make assumptions about their capacity.

In the case of a vulnerable adult (e.g., a patient with learning disability), however, judging their capacity to make a particular decision can be complex and a matter of balancing freedom with protection. Second opinions and advice are often required. Vulnerable patients may appear to have the capacity to make a decision which would potentially expose them to harm, but clinicians should maintain the principles of patient-centred care during this process (see Box 3.7).

The one situation in which clinicians are expected to act in a 'paternalistic' way is in emergencies. Unless a patient has made an advance decision which is legally binding, if consent and capacity cannot be established the clinician is required to act in the best interests of the patient.

Mrs James, a 36-year-old with severe cerebral palsy had a recent hospital admission. She was diagnosed with delirium due to a urinary tract infection. Her general practitioners are concerned that she is refusing to take her medication or to eat. She is adamant that she will not move into more supportive accommodation. She is assessed by a consultant psychiatrist as having fluctuating capacity. It is judged that missing her medication for several days will not lead to serious harm. It is a complex situation and the team decide to revisit to reassess her capacity on another occasion.

Reflective practice

Reflective practice is a vital aspect of good clinical care. One definition is that reflection is seeing our own practice through different lenses – through the literature, through the eyes of our colleagues, and the eyes of our patients. Reflection translates clinical experience into learning.

Donald Schön described four types of reflection: before action; in action; on action; and for action (see Box 3.8). Gibbs 'reflective cycle' is often used by healthcare professionals as a tool for reflection (see Figure 3.1).

Box 3.8 **Schön on reflection.**

Four types of reflection defining professionals' behaviour:

Type of reflection	Example
Reflection before action	Reflective planning before you start a task
Reflection in action	Adapting your behaviour intuitively in the middle of a clinical event such as a consultation
Reflection on action	Retrospectively thinking about actions that have already taken place
Reflection for action	Defining new goals for action, such as at an appraisal

Adapted from Schön, D.A. (1983) *The Reflective Practitioner: How professionals think in action*. Temple Smith, London.

From the start of clinical training we are taught about the importance of reflection. Students are set essays, maintain portfolios, participate in case-based discussions, look at significant events and reflect on complaints. Reflection is the backbone of appraisal and revalidation. Reflection on feedback from colleagues and patients can enable us to be more patient-centred.

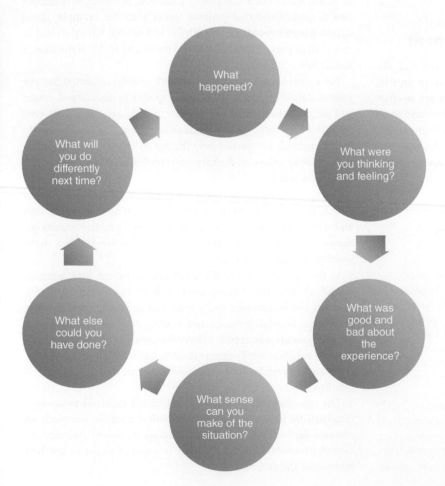

Figure 3.1 Gibbs' reflective cycle. Adapted from Gibbs, G. (1988) *Learning by Doing: A guide to teaching and learning methods*. Oxford Further Education Unit, Oxford.

Values-based practice

Values-based practice is defined as 'blending the values of both the service user and the health and social care professional, thus creating a true, as opposed to a tokenistic, partnership' (Thomas, M., 2010).

This might appear at odds with an evidence-based medicine approach, but values-based medicine should be seen as a partner. It strives to be patient-centred while acknowledging that our values and those of the patient have will an impact on the interaction. Box 3.9 lists the 10 principles of values-based practice, which overlap those of patient-centred care (Fulford, K.W.M., 2004). The 'two-feet principle' reminds us that all decisions stand on two feet, on both evidence and values, with the 'squeaky wheel principle' suggesting that we only start to see the values when the problem is contentious. Take a moment to reflect on your own values.

It is worth reflecting on our own values. They could be universal such as kindness, honesty and altruism. Certain values such as punctuality, believing in infection control and confidentiality may tie in with our professionalism. Other values may have a negative impact on our care, such as focussing on income or clock-watching. These values might result in not tolerating patients who do not follow our advice, prevent us from meeting financial targets, or finding we cannot take time to properly explain the pros and cons of a treatment as we feel we always need to finish promptly.

Fostering patient-centred care

Authors Peter and Liz Tate (see Further reading/resources) suggest that practising patient-centred care, in principle, is not difficult. It can be simply a matter of listening, being curious and having a dialogue rather than a monologue. Overall you really have to want to do it. They ask, 'Do we want to do this enough to become good at it?', and explore the idea that attitude is a key part of patient-centred care. One of the reasons they feel change has been so slow is that clinicians do not feel that patient-centred care, shared decision making and evidence-based medicine are worth the time and effort that we need to take in order to get good at it. They propose a series of questions to ask yourself after an interaction (see Box 3.10).

The Tates suggest that fostering patient-centred care, like any area of our work as a professional, needs to be learned, practised and performed.

Shared decision-making

Shared decision making embodies patient-centred care and places the beliefs, values and wishes of the patient at the centre of decision-making, although it has been described as rarely happening, hard to do and not taught. Tuckett describes shared decision-making as a meeting of experts – the patient an expert in their own life, health and beliefs with the doctor an expert in medicine (Tuckett, D. *et al.*, 1985).

Some 75% of patients wish to be involved in their health decisions, yet many are not, and this mismatch causes anxiety. Less than half of doctors follow guidelines in the USA, and similarly only half of patients are compliant with treatment. The 'Choosing wisely'

Box 3.9 **The 10 principles of values-based practice.**

Practice skills
1 Awareness
2 Reasoning
3 Knowledge
4 Communication

Modules of service delivery
5 User-centred
6 Multi-disciplinary

Values-based practice and evidence-based practice
7 The two-feet principle
8 The squeaky wheel principle
9 Science and values
10 Partnership

Adapted from Fulford, K.W.M. (2004) Ten principles of values-based medicine. In: J. Radden (ed.), *The Philosophy of Psychiatry: A Companion.* Oxford University Press, New York.
Reproduced from Thistlethwaite, J. and McKimm, J. (eds) (2015) *Health Care Professionalism at a Glance.* Wiley-Blackwell, Oxford.

Box 3.10 **Questions to ask yourself after an interaction.**

1 Do I know significantly more about this patient than I did before they came through the door?
2 Was I curious?
3 Did I really listen?
4 Did I find out what really mattered to them?
5 Did I explore their agenda, including their beliefs and expectations?
6 Did I make an acceptable working diagnosis?
7 Did I use what they thought when I started explaining?
8 Did I give them the opportunity to be involved in the decision?
9 Did I explore their understanding of the treatment?
10 Did I make some attempt to check that they really understood?
11 Did we agree on (1) the diagnosis, (2) the management, (3) the follow up?
12 Have I recorded the salient information?
13 Was I friendly?
14 Did I do this in an appropriate timescale?

Source: Tate, P. and Tate, L. (2014) *The Doctor's Communication Handbook.* Radcliffe, London. (permission requested).

campaign advises patients to ask five questions of their clinician (http://www.choosingwisely.co.uk/i-am-a-patient-carer/questions-ask-doctor). (see Box 3.11).

Shared-decision making can be difficult with vulnerable patients. Certain groups of patients are considered particularly vulnerable; these include people with mental illness, frail older people, addicts and prisoners.

As clinicians, we are in a responsible position to ensure that our vulnerable patients' needs are addressed and that their disadvantages

Box 3.11 **Five questions a patient should ask their clinician. as suggested by the 'choose wisely' campaign.**

- Do I really need this test, treatment or procedure?
- What are the risks or downsides?
- What are the possible side effects?
- Are there simpler, safer options?
- What will happen if I do nothing?

Source: http://www.choosingwisely.co.uk/i-am-a-patient-carer/questions-ask-doctor/ (accessed April 2017).

are negated. We should not make assumptions about their needs or wishes.

Patient-centred care might require health delivery to be reconsidered, for example, through outreach clinics in communities to bring healthcare to the homeless, or a flexible approach to missed appointments by patients with mental health problems.

Conclusions

Patient-centred care and whole-person care are terms that remind us to integrate medical and patient perspectives and to look at our patients holistically. In reflecting on patient-centred care, it seems that if our attitude is right and we *want* to be patient-centred, then everything else will fall into place. We hope we will find that, unlike the oncologists questioned in 1996, we will ask our patients what their needs, fears, hopes, ideas and expectations are, without finding ourselves unable to cope with their answers.

We can be prepared, with knowledge and aids, to share decisions with our patients. We can pay more attention to the needs of our most vulnerable patients to ensure that the issues they need to discuss and the symptoms they are afraid to tell us are explored.

For most clinicians, the reason we work is to care for patients. This is often challenging, but taking time often saves time down the line, and a patient-centred approach leads to better outcomes.

Further reading/resources

Kalanathi, P. (2016) *When Breath Becomes Air*. Bodley Head, London.

Ballatt, J. and Campling, P. (2011) *Intelligent kindness, reforming the culture of healthcare*. RCPsych Publications, London.

Cooper, N. and Frain, J. (eds) (2017) *ABC of Clinical Communication*. Wiley, Oxford.

British Medical Association (2012) *Medical ethics today. The BMA Handbook of Ethics and Law*. Wiley-Blackwell, Oxford.

Thomas, M., Burt, M. and Parkes, J. (2010) The Emergence of Evidence-based Practice, in *Values-Based Health & Social Care: Beyond Evidence-Based Practice* (eds J. McCarthy and P. Rose), Chapter 1, Sage, London.

Tate, P. and Tate, L. (2014) *The Doctor's Communication Handbook*. Radcliffe, London.

Tuckett, D., Boulton, M., Olson, C. and Williams. A. (1985) *Meetings between Experts. An Approach to Sharing Ideas in Medical Consultations*. Routledge, New York.

Thistlethwaite, J. and McKimm, J. (eds) (2015) *Health Care Professionalism at a Glance*. Wiley-Blackwell, Oxford.

Choosing wisely campaign: http://www.choosingwisely.co.uk/i-am-a-patient-carer/questions-ask-doctor.

CHAPTER 4

Burnout and Resilience

Clare Gerada

Medical Director Practitioner Health Programme, Riverside Medical Centre, London, UK

> ### OVERVIEW
>
> - Burnout is common, but can be managed.
> - Burnout could be considered to be an occupational hazard for all doctors.
> - There is overlap between resilience and burnout.
> - Factors such as friends, time out and mentorship replenish well-being, and addressing these can help manage or avoid burnout.
> - Systemic issues such as unreasonable workload and professional isolation can lead to burnout and should be addressed.

Definitions

While those who use the term 'burnout' know what they are trying to convey, there is in fact no standardised definition. This is important when it comes to trying to research the subject. The term was created by the psychologist Herbert Freudenberger in 1974, when he described job dissatisfaction precipitated by work-related stress. Rather than a single disorder or syndrome, burnout should be considered a spectrum of symptoms ranging from physical and/or emotional exhaustion impacting on the individual's ability to work: tearfulness, depersonalisation, depression and anxiety. The Maslach Burnout Inventory (MBI) (see Further reading/resources) has been used for around 25 years to measure burnout in three domains:

- Emotional exhaustion: measures feelings of being emotionally overextended and exhausted by one's work.
- Depersonalisation: measures an unfeeling and impersonal response to those who receive the individual's services, treatment or instruction.
- Personal accomplishment: measures feelings of competence and successful achievement in one's work.

The World Health Organization International Classification of Diseases (10th revision) defines burnout as a 'state of vital exhaustion'.

Whichever definition is used, those who describe themselves as 'burnt out', or those who score on rating scales for burnout, have a range of physical (headaches, insomnia, gastrointestinal disturbances) and psychological (low mood, anxiety, irritability, decreased concentration) symptoms. Burnout can lead to depression and contribute to job dissatisfaction, marital difficulties and impact on the ability to work effectively, leading (for healthcare professionals) to errors, poor patient satisfaction and lower quality of care. Burnout is more common among those in the caring professions – especially in those where there is a high degree of altruism, vocational spirit and making others (namely patients) their main concern (see Figure 4.1).

Resilience

All healthcare professionals, in particular doctors, must be resilient if they are to survive long and gruelling training and the constant exposure to death, distress and disability. They need to be adaptable and flexible, able to absorb the pressures of work, and build psychological defences to cope with the stresses of medicine and the ethical and moral challenges associated with being a modern doctor. These defences act as a necessary barrier to the emotions which are generated when dealing with illness, and act to protect health professionals from burn out. Doctors need the ability to not only survive, but also to thrive and adapt in the face of adversity; to be committed, persistent and confident in their ability and remain compassionate with patients.

As with individuals, organisations have degrees of resilience such that they can survive enormous organisational change or trauma. For example, it is impossible to escape structural, managerial or service delivery change – nothing stands still in time. Organisations with a culture of openness, good lines of communication and systems to address staff concerns help to contain the inevitable anxiety created by change.

Resilience is always contextual; a complex and dynamic interplay between the individual, their environment and sociocultural factors, and any intervention into promoting resilience must address organisational as well as individual and team issues. This means that classroom teaching for resilience is unlikely to be effective unless followed up by changes in the working environment. No amount of classroom training can compensate for persistent poor

---

ABC of Clinical Professionalism, First Edition. Edited by Nicola Cooper, Anna Frain and John Frain.
© 2018 John Wiley & Sons Ltd. Published 2018 by John Wiley & Sons Ltd.

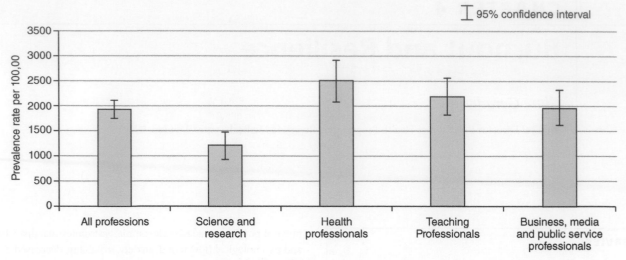

Figure 4.1 Prevalence rate of work-related stress within the category of all professions per 100 000 people employed averaged over the period 2011/12, 2013/14 and 2014/15. Reproduced from the UK Government's Health and Safety Executive (open access) www.hse.gov.uk/statistics/lfs/strocc2_3yr.xlsx.

working conditions. Addressing these conditions and putting in place practical measures to improve working lives and reduce workload would do more to improve health and well-being than any amount of 'resilience training'.

In general, burnout is due to a combination of:

- Internal resources, vulnerabilities and coping mechanisms.
- Organisational factors, including work pressure, resources (time, people and money) and spaces and opportunities for team working.
- Environmental and external factors, including regulatory requirements, political influences, media pressures.

Resilience and mental health disorders

Resilience is not simply the absence of burnout, but burnout might represent an end stage of failed resilience and make it more difficult to plan early interventions to increase resilience. There is a considerable overlap between resilience and burnout, and also to concepts such as 'wellness and well-being'. Wellness, described as the complete mental, physical and emotional well-being of an individual, is a characteristic that can increase resilience, and resilience is a component of well-being. The opposite of wellness is illness, and the opposite of burnout is full engagement. Small improvements in well-being or reducing risk factors across the whole population would reduce the number of people developing mental illness. Improving mental well-being can improve an individual's physical health and reduce mortality.

Medical students and burnout

Burnout is prevalent among the medical profession, with rates increasing during training and after qualification. A 2006 study conducted by Rosen *et al.* (see Further reading/resources) of American doctors showed that at the beginning of the intern year, 4.3% of internal medicine residents met criteria for burnout, as measured by the MBI. By the end of the first year the rates had increased to 55.3%, with a significant increase in both the depersonalisation and

emotional exhaustion subscales. Another study of internal medicine residents at the University of Washington found that 76% met criteria for burnout as measured by the MBI, regardless of postgraduate year (Shanafelt, T.D. *et al.*, 2002). A study of UK medical students found equally high rates of burnout (as measured by the MBI) with levels across the different subscales from 55% (emotional exhaustion), 34% (depersonalization) and 47% (personal accomplishment) (Cecil, J. *et al.*, 2014). The same study also examined lifestyle factors such as alcohol use and exercise. The study concluded that burnout was a significant issue in undergraduate medical students in the UK, and health behaviours – particularly physical activity – predict components of burnout. Gender, year of study and institution also appear to influence the prevalence of burnout. Encouraging medical students to make healthier lifestyle choices early in their medical training may reduce the likelihood of the development of burnout. Exercise can help to improve the symptoms of burnout amongst medical students. In addition, the UK medical student study indicated that specific demographic, lifestyle and behavioural factors, including physical activity, sweet or savoury food consumption, alcohol bingeing, gender, year and institution of study, may predict medical students' experience of burnout components, although the amount of variance in burnout predicted by these health behaviours is small. Willcock *et al.* (see Further reading/resources), showed that, during the transition from final-year medical students to first year of training, the point prevalence of burnout steadily increased.

Professional distress

Since 2008 the NHS Practitioner Health Programme (PHP; www.php.nhs.uk) has been providing a confidential service to doctors and dentists with mental health and/or addiction problems. The service was established following the suicide of a young psychiatrist who, before killing herself, also killed her three-month-old baby. The subsequent inquiry identified the high rates of mental illness among the medical profession coupled with low rates of access to treatment – with many doctors presenting late in their illness, usually following a crisis at work or a drink-drive offence. A review of the mental health of doctors provided evidence to suggest that doctors have increased rates of burnout, mental health problems, substance misuse and suicide rates compared to other professionals and the general population.

Mental illness in doctors is a global phenomenon. In UK studies it has been suggested that 10–20% of all doctors become depressed at some point in their lives, and have a higher suicide rate than the general population. There is some evidence that mental illness is increasing, especially amongst younger doctors. For example, over a six-year period the age of doctors presenting to the PHP decreased from an average of 44 years to 37 years, with over 50% of the cohort presenting in 2015 aged under 35 years. This is in keeping with trends found in other services for training-grade doctors.

The 7th National GP Work Life Survey Report 2012, from the University of Manchester, examined over time the working conditions of general practitioners and attitudes to primary care during major health service reforms in England. In 2012, the key findings were:

- Lowest level job satisfaction since 2001.
- Increase in hours of work.
- Reported levels of stress highest since beginning of National GP Work Life Survey series in 1998.
- The proportion of GPs expecting to quit increased from 6.4% in 2010 to 8.9% in 2012 amongst GPs aged under 50 years old, and from 41.7% in 2010 to 54.1% in 2012 amongst GPs aged 50 years and over.

From January 2017, the General Practitioner Health Service (GPHS) has been in operation in England. This extends the current practitioner health service and means that around 85 000 doctors can access confidential physician health services. This service will provide similar services to PHP, as well as a focus on prevention, through psychoeducation, group work and self help material. Doctors presenting to the new GPH are unwell, primarily with mental health issues rather than addiction. They fall into four main groups:

- A struggling practice, with one individual left holding the fort, now becoming unwell themselves.
- A complaint or investigation has led to a breakdown in mental health.
- Younger doctors unable to cope with the pressure and strains of the role.
- An individual who has become mentally unwell, leading to a mistake or error.

The impact of burnout on patients

Mental illness among doctors matters, not just to them (as patients) but also to the patients they treat. Doctors who suffer from health problems, such as stress and substance abuse, were found to have been performing at a suboptimal level for some time before they 'burn out' (see Box 4.1).

For example, a study of American surgeons suffering from psychological distress with poor mental quality of life, symptoms of depression and burnout were found to report an increased number of major medical errors compared to those with low levels of psychological distress (Shanafelt, T.D., *et al.*, 2010). Similarly, studies have shown that where doctors have high levels of fatigue they report more medical errors. A study into patient satisfaction in primary care in Greece reported decreased levels of patient

Box 4.1 **Examples illustrating the development of burnout.**

Case 1

Jane had just qualified and was starting her first foundation year post. She was now in her second week and finding things very different from medical school. She felt unsupported, always out of her depth, and was constantly asking for help, but feeling very guilty about it. She seemed to have forgotten all that she had learnt and began to doubt her career choice.

Even though she was not yet doing night work she began even to worry about this – if she couldn't cope within normal working hours, how would she be able to cope out of hours? She began staying longer and longer at work, constantly checking what she was doing was right. She even started coming in on her days off 'just to make sure'.

She found that she was irritable with her boyfriend and dreaded time off in case one of her 'errors would be found out when she was away'. After a difficult handover she couldn't stop crying and approached her consultant for help.

Case 2

Dr Brown had worked in his practice for 23 years. He had recently been made senior partner as two of his partners had recently taken early retirement. Another of his partners was on maternity leave, and yet another on sick leave following a fractured leg.

He found it difficult to get help in the practice and was working increasingly long hours to meet all the demands that his patients and his practice made on him. Once home he would also log into the practice system and finish the results and letters.

He found that he was drinking more coffee to stay awake and finding it difficult to get to sleep, lying for hours worrying about his work. After one particularly long and difficult Monday morning surgery he felt he couldn't go on any more, feeling that he had failed his patients.

satisfaction of consultations with doctors with higher levels of burnout (Anagnostopoulos, F. and Niakas, D., *et al.*, 2012).

Causes of distress

The rise in distress amongst doctors is a global issue. The causes of this are likely to be multifactorial. There are a number of risk factors which either alone or through their interaction might increase the likelihood of doctors becoming ill, and then once unwell prevent them from seeking appropriate help (see Box 4.2).

There are other external factors to the rising levels of mental distress among health professionals. Medicine and those who work in the health system are in a state of flux as the way care is delivered is being industrialised and privatised – changing and in many ways damaging the doctor/nurse–patient relationship. For doctors in particular, their training, with its multi-professional focus, non-medically led hierarchies and loss of 'medical spaces' such as the Doctors Mess or doctor-only dining room, no longer permit such close identification with each other. Once qualified, loss of the traditional (medical) 'firm' and new complex rotas mean that there is little continuity in terms of stable teams, wards, or even hospitals for doctors in training. A doctor is also unlikely to be able to follow

Box 4.2 **Risk factors which might increase the likelihood of doctors becoming ill.**

Risk factors

Occupational (related to the job)	
Clinical	Emotional demands of working with patients and working so close to death, despair and disability.
	High expectations about the power of medicine putting unrealistic pressure on doctors.
	Easy access to prescription drugs and knowledge of how to use them.
Structural	Heavy workload and long and unpredictable working hours.
	Sleep deprivation.
	Psychosocial work environment such as workplace bullying; and lack of cohesive teamwork and social support, leading them to work individually, whereas working in teams is associated with being better able to cope with stress.
Individual	
Personality and psychological vulnerabilities	Defences, such as depersonalisation and denial of feelings are necessary to work in close proximity to death, despair and disease. But if left unchecked, these can act as barriers to getting help and lead instead to doctors working harder rather than taking time off work.
	Personality traits – common in good doctors, if exaggerated can cause problems, including:
	• Denigration of vulnerability 'I care for others more than I care for myself';
	• Narcissism: 'I must be the best';
	• Perfectionism: 'I must do this right and mistakes are intolerable in me or others';
	• Compulsiveness: 'I have to do this, and I can't give up till I finish'.
	Firth-Cozens makes the point that the difficult and emotionally demanding job of a doctor frequently leads to doctors being self-critical.
	Other psychological vulnerabilities common in physicians have been identified, including an excessive sense of responsibility, desire to please everyone, guilt for things outside of one's own control, self-doubt and obsessive compulsive traits.
Barriers to seeking help	
Physical and practical	Frequent changes of address make it difficult to build up a sustaining relationship with a GP or Mental Health Service.
	Concerns as to career if time spent seeking help for mental health problems.
	Doctors report high levels of 'presenteeism' (attending work even when not feeling well enough to do so).
	Concerns about confidentiality.
	Concerns that disclosure of mental illness might require regulatory involvement (GMC) which could lead to a long period of stress and confusion due to the lengthy investigations that take place when doctors are suspended.
Psychological	Feelings of shame and embarrassment.
	Pressure for doctors to appear healthy.
	Doctors may see illness as a mark of failure.
	Doctors find it difficult to take on the 'patient role' linked to their training and over-identification with the 'caring' role.
	Even when becoming patients, other doctors treat them differently.
Systemic	Under-funding.
	Over-reliance on inspection.
	Constant reorganisation.
	Industrialisation of healthcare.

the care of their patient throughout their stay in hospital, creating dissatisfaction for doctor and patient alike.

Support mechanisms

Most doctor-directed interventions involve mindfulness, behavioural treatment, mentoring, coaching or addressing personal coping strategies, and the evidence shows that, irrespective of the modality, the outcome is the same – improvement in attention.

A good conceptual model of reducing the risk of burnout has been devised by Dunn *et al.* (see Further reading/resources) (see Figure 4.2).

This illustrates positive and negative factors which influence the development of burnout. The model considers emotional well-being to be a fixed resource, increased by positive factors such as supports, mentorship and outside interests, and depleted by negative factors such as work pressure, personal stresses and lack of time to rest. A state of well-being versus burnout is determined by the balance between these factors. It behoves each individual to identify personal factors which can have a negative or positive impact on well-being, for example:

• Ensuring that one takes all allocated annual leave.
• Engaging in hobbies.
• Maintaining social networks.

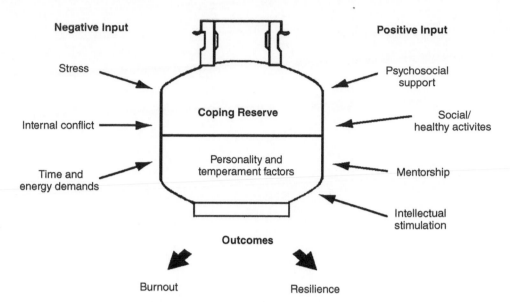

Figure 4.2 Conceptual model of reducing the risk of burnout – The Coping Reserve Tank. A conceptual model of medical student well- being the 'Coping Reserve Tank'. Reproduced with permission from Dunn, L.B., Iglewicz, A. and Moutier C. (2008) A conceptual model of medical student well-being: promoting resilience and preventing burnout. *Academic Psychiatry*, **32** (1), 44–53.

- Engaging in a reflective practice (e.g., a Balint group).
- Mentors/coaching.

Balme and Gerada (see Further reading/resources) have reviewed different factors associated with the development of mental health problems among doctors. Not surprisingly, the risks of burnout are reduced if doctors (and medical students) take time out, have interests outside medicine, have family or other support networks, take regular exercise and have a sense of humour. Research shows that simple interventions such as taking holidays, having time with friends or family, sport, music or simply just standing still helps to reduce burnout. For each health professional it is important to realise their limits and when things appear to be going wrong, or their mood dips or they begin to resort to unhealthy coping strategies, then they need to think about seeking help.

The author has designed an acronym to summarise the ways of reducing the risk of burnout (see Box 4.3).

Conclusions

Burnout is common, and a normal aspect of a healthcare professional's work. Going forward, healthcare professionals – and doctors in particular – have to learn to identify it and manage it throughout their professional lives.

Further reading/resources

For information as to where to get support for mental health problems and/or burnout, see: www.php.nhs.uk; or www.gphealth.nhs.uk; or https://www.bma.org.uk/advice/work-life-support/your-wellbeing/doctor-support-service.

Anagnostopoulos, F. and Niakas, D. (2012) Job burnout, health-related quality of life, and sickness absence in Greek health professionals. *Journal of Clinical Psychology in Medical Settings*, **19** (4), 401–410

Balme, E. and Gerada, C. (2016) *The vital signs in primary care. A guide for GPs seeking help and advice*. Royal Medical Benevolent Fund. Available at: http://rmbf.org/wp-content/uploads/2017/01/rmbf-the-vital-signs-in-primary-care.pdf.

Cecil, J., McHale, C., Hart, J. and Laidlaw, A. (2014) Behaviour and burnout in medical students. *Medical Education Online*, **19**, 10.3402/meo.v19.25209. DOI: 10.3402/meo.v19.25209.

Dunn, L.B., Iglewicz, A. and Moutier, C. (2008) A conceptual model of medical student wellbeing: promoting resilience and preventing burnout. *Academic Psychiatry*, **32** (1), 44–53

Maslach, C. (1993) Burnout: a multidimensional perspective, in *Professional Burnout: Recent Developments in Theory and Research*. (eds W.B. Schaufeli, C. Maslach and T. Marek), Taylor & Francis, Washington, DC. https://www.statisticssolutions.com/maslach-burnout-inventory-mbi/

Rosen, I.M., Gimotty, P.A. and Shea, J.A. (2006) Evolution of sleep quantity, sleep deprivation, mood disturbances, empathy and burnout among interns. *Academic Medicine*, **81** (1), 82–85.

Shanafelt, T.D., Bradley, K.A., Wipf, J.E. and Back, A.L. (2002) Burnout and self reported patient care in an internal medicine residency program. *Annals of Internal Medicine*, **136** (5), 358–367.

Willcock, S.M., Daly, M.G., Tennant, C.C. and Allard, B.J. (2004) Burnout and psychiatric morbidity in new medical graduates. *Medical Journal of Australia*, **181** (7), 357–360. http://www.blmc.co.uk/docs/Doctors%20in%20difficulties_The%20Vital%20Signs%20in%20Primary%20Care.pdf (accessed April 2017).

Box 4.3 **B.U.R.N.O.U.T – an acronym to prevent burnout.**

- **B**alance work and play – between the machinery of caring and actual caring, declutter the space in the consulting room between us and our patients).
- **U**nderstand our limitations – we are not superheros.
- **R**ecognise – prevent and treat burnout in ourselves and our teams.
- **N**urture the next generation – bring the fun back in to work.
- **T**eam work – working in groups, restore the times and spaces to work, rest, play and reflect together.

CHAPTER 5

Confidentiality and Social Media

John Spandorfer

Jefferson Medical College, Philadelphia, USA

OVERVIEW

- The tenet of confidentiality is one of the most important in medicine and is grounded in oaths, codes and laws.
- Social media is increasingly used by healthcare students and professionals; social media users need to be mindful of its risks.
- When writing information about patients on social media without their authorisation, one should be aware of legal standards and ethical principles prior to posting.
- Students and healthcare professionals should be aware of policies and statements from relevant organisations on the subject of social media use.

Confidentiality – background

The tenet of patient confidentiality has been a long-held precept in medicine, inspired by oaths and more recently guided by professional codes and regulated by laws. The Hippocratic Oath (see Box 5.1) composed in the 4th century BCE by the Greek physician Hippocrates, included the obligation for physicians to maintain patient confidentiality: '*What I may see or hear in the course of the treatment or even outside of the treatment in regard to the life of men, which on no account one must spread abroad, I will keep to myself, holding such things shameful to be spoken about*'.

The 2002 Physician Charter, initiated by the European Federation of Internal Medicine, the American Board of Internal Medicine and the American College of Physicians, and later endorsed by medical societies worldwide, includes in its professional responsibilities the commitment to patient confidentiality. The Charter states: 'Earning the trust and confidence of patients requires that appropriate confidentiality safeguards be applied to disclosure of patient information. This commitment extends to discussions with persons acting on a patient's behalf when obtaining the patient's own consent is not feasible'.

The UK's General Medical Council guidance on confidentiality notes that: 'Confidentiality is central to trust between doctors and patients. Without assurances about confidentiality, patients may be

---

Box 5.1 The Hippocratic Oath (modern version).

I swear by Apollo Physician and Asclepiusand Hygieia and Panaceia and all the gods and goddesses, making them my witnesses, that I will fulfil according to my ability and judgment this oath and this covenant:

To hold him who has taught me this art as equal to my parents and to live my life in partnership with him, and if he is in need of money to give him a share of mine, and to regard his offspring as equal to my brothers in male lineage and to teach them this art — if they desire to learn it — without fee and covenant; to give a share of precepts and oral instruction and all the other learning to my sons and to the sons of him who has instructed me and to pupils who have signed the covenant and have taken an oath according to the medical law, but to no one else.

I will apply dietetic measures for the benefit of the sick according to my ability and judgment; I will keep them from harm and injustice.

I will neither give a deadly drug to anybody if asked for it, nor will I make a suggestion to this effect. Similarly I will not give to a woman an abortive remedy. In purity and holiness I will guard my life and my art.

I will not use the knife, not even on sufferers from stone, but will withdraw in favour of such men as are engaged in this work.

Whatever houses I may visit, I will come for the benefit of the sick, remaining free of all intentional injustice, of all mischief and in particular of sexual relations with both female and male persons, be they free or slaves.

What I may see or hear in the course of the treatment or even outside of the treatment in regard to the life of men, which on no account one must spread abroad, I will keep to myself holding such things shameful to be spoken about.

If I fulfil this oath and do not violate it, may it be granted to me to enjoy life and art, being honoured with fame among all men for all time to come; if I transgress it and swear falsely, may the opposite of all this be my lot.

Translated from the Greek by Ludwig Edelstein (1092–1965). From The Hippocratic Oath: Text, Translation and Interpretation by Ludwig Edelstein. The John Hopkins, Baltimore, 1943.

Adapted forms of the Hippocratic Oath, including the section on confidentiality, are still administered today in medical schools worldwide.

ABC of Clinical Professionalism, First Edition. Edited by Nicola Cooper, Anna Frain and John Frain.
© 2018 John Wiley & Sons Ltd. Published 2018 by John Wiley & Sons Ltd.

reluctant to seek medical attention or to give doctors the information they need in order to provide good care'. The UK's Nursing and Midwifery Council, and the Health and Care Professions Council have similar codes of confidentiality.

Laws such as the US Health Insurance Portability and Accountability Act (HIPAA; issued in 1996) and the subsequent Privacy Rule (issued in 2003) protect patient confidentiality.

Confidentiality is not absolute, however. Healthcare providers may disclose confidential medical information without the patient's permission when such disclosure is permissible by Law (e.g., giving information post-mortem to the Coroner) or for the protection of the public or specific at-risk individuals (e.g., information given to the Police relating to terrorism or given to public health officials or individuals at risk concerning a patient with specific communicable diseases such as tuberculosis).

Social media – background

Social media or Web 2.0 internet-based applications allow users to generate content and have interactive dialogues with other users. Various types of social media are listed in Box 5.2.

Increasingly medical students, doctors and other healthcare professionals are using these sites and others for personal and professional purposes. A survey of more than 4000 physicians found that 90% use social media for personal reasons and 65% for professional reasons.

Box 5.2 **Types of social media.**

Type of social media	Examples
Social networking	Facebook, LinkedIn, Sermo, Doctors.net.uk, WhatsApp, Snapchat, Instagram
Video hosting	YouTube, Vimeo
Social news	Reddit, Slashdot, Fark, Digg, Newsvine
Blogging or microblogging	Twitter, Kevin MD, lifeinthefastlane.com

Benefits and risks of social media use for clinicians

This section will focus on concerns surrounding confidentiality and social media use. However, before considering these concerns, the benefits and risks (other than confidentiality) of social media use for clinicians will be briefly mentioned. In the UK's General Medical Council Guidance, 'Doctors and Social Media' (see Figure 5.1), the authors note many areas of benefits to using social media including: (i) the rapid dissemination of new developments, ideas, position statements and upcoming meetings; (ii) collective sourcing of advice on challenging medical cases; and (iii) the ability of professional organisations to connect with its members. The authors of the

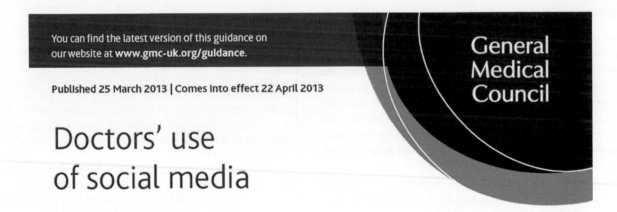

You can find the latest version of this guidance on our website at **www.gmc-uk.org/guidance**.

Published 25 March 2013 | Comes into effect 22 April 2013

Doctors' use of social media

General Medical Council

Figure 5.1 GMC Guidance on Doctors' Use of Social Media. From www.gmc-uk.org/guidance/ethical_guidance/21186.asp.
In 'Good Medical Practice' we say:

You must treat colleagues fairly and with respect
You must make sure that your conduct justifies your patients' trust in you and the public's trust in the profession
When communicating publicly, including speaking to or writing in the media, you must maintain patient confidentiality. You should remember when using social media that communications intended for friends or family may become more widely available.
When advertising your services, you must make sure the information you publish is factual and can be checked, and does not exploit patients' vulnerability of lack of knowledge.
In 'Confidentiality' we say:
Many improper disclosures are unintentional. You should not share identifiable information about patients where you can be overheard, for example in a public place or an internet chat forum.
In this guidance, we explain how doctors can put these principles in to practice [in social media]. Serious or persistent failure to follow this guidance will put your registration at risk.
From www.gmc-uk.org/guidance/ethical_guidance/21186.asp (accessed February 2017).

guidance also take note of risks. These include: (i) potential doctor–patient boundary violations (e.g., 'friending' on Facebook); and (ii) the potential for undermining patients' trust in the doctor, particularly if the doctor posts a story or photograph that may be perceived as being unprofessional.

Confidentiality violations on social media – prevalence

In a 2012 US survey of all state medical boards about online professionalism violations, 60% reported receiving notification of at least one violation of online patient confidentiality. In a review of social media use among clinicians, von Muhlen and Ohno-Machado noted the small but growing number of confidentiality violations among Facebook- and Twitter-using medical students and doctors. These and other authors noted the expectation that these violations will continue to rise as the use of social media grows.

Confidentiality violations on social media – examples

The following examples illustrate some common confidentiality violations on social media:

- A resident posted to his social media site a photograph that was of him being hugged by his patient. The photo, taken by a nurse and emailed to the resident, was of the patient at the time of discharge and followed a prolonged hospitalisation that involved a heart transplant. Below the photograph he wrote. 'So excited and proud to be involved! Almost one year waiting and now a new heart and going home!'
- A fourth-year medical student on an Emergency Medicine rotation was on the trauma team that cared for two patients who were involved in a motor vehicle collision. One patient died of his injuries, the other survived. That evening, the student posted on her social media site a photo taken of the X-ray of the femur fracture of the surviving patient. The name on the photo was redacted. In addition to posting the photo, the student wrote: 'Sad story from the ED last night. Two passengers in an MVC. One dead on arrival, the other with multiple fractures, including this fracture. No one wearing seatbelts. Ugh!'
- A physician made the following post on his social media site: 'It never ceases to amaze me how people can get so fat. And it's getting worse! I'll never forget the incredibly obese woman who nearly got stuck in the CT scanner and the other even larger one who almost broke the stretcher. We should ship these folks to an animal hospital where they can handle massive patients!'

Confidentiality violations – legal, professional and ethical considerations

While considering whether a social media post is a violation of confidentiality, it is useful to consider whether the post violates a standard of legal conduct or more generally violates a standard of professional or ethical conduct. In the US, the Health Insurance Portability and Accountability Act (HIPAA), issued in 1996, and the subsequent Privacy Rule, issued in 2003, protect patient confidentiality. The HIPAA statute notes that, 'There are no restrictions on the use or disclosure of de-identified health information. De-identified health information neither identifies nor provides a reasonable basis to identify an individual'. The following excerpt from HIPAA describes the process of de-identifying medical information:

'There are two ways to de-identify information: (1) a formal determination by a qualified statistician; and (2) the removal of specified identifiers of an individual and of the individual's relatives, household members, and employers, and is adequate only if the covered entity has no actual knowledge that the remaining information could be used to identify the individual'.

The UK National Health Service's confidentiality policy, issued in 2014, also stipulates that confidential information can be disclosed provided that the information is 'effectively anonymised', although it gives no specific instructions how to anonymise the information.

In the first example of confidentiality violations, although likely well-intentioned, the post of the photograph by the resident physician was inappropriate as it clearly met the legal violation threshold. Yet one can appreciate how easy it is to commit such an error. The resident's patient was discharged following a long hospitalisation and the photograph commemorates this success. He wants to share this important memory, much like other non-professional life events, with his friends who follow his social media site. Without active awareness of the significance of this privacy violation, as well as its prevention, the inadvertent merger of confidential medical information and social media may too easily occur.

In the second example, the question of a legal violation is not as clear. Although there was no name on the radiograph, a reader of the post who both knew where the student was doing her Emergency Medicine rotation and had heard of the unique event (the recent accident leading to a fatality), may be able to identify the patient with the fractured femur. Prior to posting the radiograph and text, the student should have deduced that one of the 'followers' of her post could have the ability, if motivated, to identify the patient. The risk of violating patient confidentiality when posting a story on social media, where the numbers of followers may be high, are significantly greater than verbally telling the same story to a far more limited number of listeners. Had the medical student shared this story with an old friend who lived in another part of the country, the risk of that friend identifying the victim would have been exceedingly low, and it may have met the HIPAA criteria of de-identification if the student had 'no actual knowledge that the remaining information could be used to identify the individual'.

In the third example, the information posted by the physician complaining about his obese patients appears to include no identifying information and therefore would not be a violation of HIPAA or other legal standards. It would however be a professional and ethical violation, and likely a violation of the physician's hospital or health system code of conduct. Any post that disparages or ridicules patients erodes the trust that readers would have in that physician. In the first line of the Physician Charter, it is written that, 'Professionalism is the basis of medicine's contract with society. Essential to this contract is public trust in physicians which depends on the integrity of both individual physicians and the whole profession'. Furthermore, the Charter states that, 'Professionalism demands placing the interest of patients above those of the physician'. This post by the physician violates key aspects of professional behaviour. It shows a clear lack of integrity and places the interest of the physician, who appears to be venting his frustration, over the interests of the patients he is ridiculing. The physician's post also undermines any patient's belief that their own privacy will be maintained, regardless of whether the post includes identifying information or violates a legal standard. And finally, the post violates the oath of Hippocrates, which states: 'What I may see or hear in the course of the treatment or even outside of the treatment in regard to the life of men, which on no account one must spread abroad, I will keep to myself, holding such things shameful to be spoken about'.

Appropriate posts on social media

If each of the examples above illustrate inappropriate social media posts, would it ever be *appropriate* to write about patients on social media? Stevenson and Peck, as well as Chretien and Kind, propose a model, using 'the double-effect' reasoning, when considering the ethics of social media posts. The authors recommend the following criteria:

- The social media post considered separately from its unintended harmful effect is in itself not wrong.
- The writer intends only the good and does not intend harm as an end or as a mean.
- The writer reflects upon his/her relevant duties, considering accepted norms and takes due care to eliminate or alleviate any foreseen harm through his/her act.

Although the physician writing about the overweight patients met none of these criteria, many respectfully written posts by healthcare providers may do so. Prior to writing on social media, patient permission should be sought. When patients are informed about the beneficial purpose of the writing and assured there would be de-identification (unless the patient chooses to be identified), they may consent to having their story written. But, as illustrated in the example of the student in the emergency room, proper de-identification requires prudence.

As suggested by Chretien and Kind, the following types of post that consider the intent of the writer meet the criteria above and may be justified; these are listed in Box 5.3.

Recommendations from professional organisations

National medical, nursing and allied health regulators have comprehensive guidance on confidentiality and social media. In addition, universities and individual healthcare organisations are likely to have their own policies that students or employees are required to follow.

General Medical Council's Good Medical Practice

'When communicating publicly, including speaking to or writing in the media, you must maintain patient confidentiality. You should remember when using social media that communications intended for friends or family may become more widely available … You should be aware of the limitations of privacy online and you should regularly review the privacy settings for each of your social media profiles. This is for the following reasons:

- Social media sites cannot guarantee confidentiality, whatever privacy settings are in place.

Box 5.3 **Examples of appropriate social media posts.**

Intent of writer	Suggested modification of social media post examples	Example post
Stimulate understanding or empathy without intention to harm.	The resident instead writes about the difficulties patients with complex problems have and how fortunate it is to be with them through and at the happy conclusion of their hospitalization.	A photo of the resident and a colleague in front of the hospital with the caption, 'We are inspired by many of our patients who have been through so much. Thrilled to be involved in their care!'
Fulfil the role of teacher.	The student instead writes at the conclusion of his or her Emergency Medicine rotation about the many injuries he/she has seen resulting from car accidents that could have been prevented by wearing seat belts.	'Until I cared for a trauma victim who wasn't buckled up, I didn't realise just how stupid it is to not to wear a seatbelt!'
Reflection about the provider's professional and ethical duties.	The physician instead writes about the challenges that morbidly obese patients have.	'After caring for several morbidly obese patients over the years, and observing their struggles in the hospital – dealing with stretchers and scanners that are too small, overhearing disparaging comments – you realise that as a profession, we've got to figure out how to make better accommodations for this patient population'.

- Patients, your employers, or any other organisation you have a relationship with, may be able to access your personal information.
- Information about your location may be embedded within photographs and other content and available for others to see.
- Once information is published online it can be difficult to remove as others may distribute it further or comment on it.'

American College of Physicians and Federation of State Medical Boards

'Use of online media can bring significant educational benefits to patients and physicians, but may also pose ethical challenges. Maintaining trust in the profession and in patient–physician relationships requires that physicians consistently apply ethical principles for preserving the relationship, confidentiality, privacy, and respect for persons to online settings and communications'.

American Medical Association

'Physicians should be cognisant of standards of patient privacy and confidentiality that must be maintained in all environments, including online, and must refrain from posting identifiable patient information online'.

Nursing and Midwifery Council (UK)

'Nurses and midwives may put their registration at risk, and students may jeopardise their ability to join our register, if they act in any way that is unprofessional or unlawful on social media including (but not limited to):
- Sharing confidential information inappropriately.
- Posting pictures of patients and people receiving care without their consent.
- Posting inappropriate comments about patients.
- Bullying, intimidating or exploiting people.
- Building or pursuing relationships with patients or service users.
- Stealing personal information or using someone else's identity.
- Encouraging violence or self-harm.
- Inciting hatred or discrimination.

If you are aware that another nurse or midwife has used social media in any of these ways, it might be helpful to refer to our guidance on raising concerns (NMC, 2013). This sets out your professional duty to report any concerns you have about the safety of people in your care or the public, and the steps you should take to do this'.

Top tips for posting on social media sites

Prior to posting on social media sites about your work or about patients, first consider if the writing or photograph contains potentially identifying information. If so, consent must be obtained prior to posting. If the writing or photograph does not contain identifying information, the post may be appropriate if it is respectfully written *and* at least one of the following criteria are met:
- When it is likely there would be an educational benefit from sharing a lesson learned during the care of the patient.
- When a post can invoke empathy or compassion for patients.
- When a post can improve the understanding of the challenges of caring for patients.
- When medical advice for a challenging medical case is needed – this would only be appropriate for a site restricted to healthcare personnel and should only include the minimum necessary information required.

Conclusions

The use of social media has many benefits, but healthcare professionals are required to adhere to rules about confidentiality as well as professional behaviour. It is sometimes easy to forget how public social media can be. Conversations are not private and can be reposted and viewed by others, with potentially serious unintended consequences. All healthcare professionals, including students, have a duty to understand their responsibilities.

Further reading/resources

ABIM Foundation. American Board of Internal Medicine (2001) ACP-ASIM Foundation. American College of Physicians-American Society of Internal Medicine; European Federation of Internal Medicine. Medical professionalism in the new millennium: a physician charter. *Annals of Internal Medicine*, **136** (3), 243–246.

American Medical Association (2017) Professionalism in the Use of Social Media, 2.3.3. www.ama-assn.org/ama/pub/physician-resources/medical-ethics/code-medical-ethics.page (accessed February 2017).

Chretien, K.C. and Kind, T. (2013) Social Media and Clinical Care. Ethical, Professional, and Social Implications. *Circulation*, **127**, 1413–1421.

Fogelson, N.S., Rubin, Z.A. and Ault, K.A. (2013) Beyond likes and tweets: an in-depth look at the physician social media landscape. *Clinical Obstetrics and Gynecology*, **56** (3), 495–508.

General Medical Council. Doctors' Use of Social Media. www.gmc-uk.org/guidance/ethical_guidance/21186.asp (accessed February 2017).

Von Muhlen, M. and Ohno-Machado, L. (2012) Reviewing social media use by clinicians. *Journal of the American Medical Informatics Association*, **19**, 777–781.

CHAPTER 6

The Culture of Healthcare

Charlotte E. Rees[1] and Lynn V. Monrouxe[2]

[1] Faculty of Medicine, Nursing and Health Sciences, Monash University, Australia
[2] Chang Gung Medical Education Research Center (CG-MERC), Chang Gung Memorial Hospital, Linkou, Taiwan

---

OVERVIEW

- Healthcare students learn the knowledge, skills, attitudes and practices of their chosen profession partly through the healthcare culture.

- The hidden curriculum relates to elements of healthcare students' socialisation into the norms, values and practices of the healthcare culture.

- We can better understand the healthcare culture through examining the physical environment, the bodies of students and staff, institutional slang and derogatory humour and intentional socialisation practices.

- Both leader- and student-driven strategies are needed to improve the healthcare culture.

Introduction

"Nurse gave an incompetent handover followed by revealing that medication had been left on [a] patient's table in her bay... My mentor was also present and saw this incident, as well as seeing the awful handover. I told my mentor it was poor practice, she agreed. I asked her what [the] procedure was for reporting the incident... and she said '*just leave it*'. I asked her to consider that we could find ourselves on this ward at some point, at the mercy of this awful care and shouldn't we deal with it? I also pointed out that we shouldn't wait for someone to be injured before taking action. I wanted to galvanise her to act. It didn't work. She had complained about this nurse before and it had come to nothing. She wasn't prepared to try again for fear of being seen as '*rocking the boat*'. I still feel bad... If poor performance is not tackled and managers cannot performance manage staff I do not feel it is the place of students, who need to be employed once qualified, to stick their necks out against [an] ingrained NHS [National Health Service] culture".

Maud, Female, Year 2, Nursing Student, UK

Healthcare culture matters: it is the complex whole through which healthcare students learn the knowledge, skills, attitudes and practices of their chosen professions in order to become fully fledged members. While students are taught professionalism through the formal curriculum underpinned by regulatory body codes of practice, much of what they learn comes from their observation of healthcare cultures as part of their workplace learning experiences. Consider Maud's narrative above: through what she calls an '*ingrained NHS culture*', she learns that poor practice exists and is normalised through its acceptance by institutional leaders, as has been found elsewhere in high-profile healthcare inquiries (e.g., Francis, 2013; see Further reading/resources). In this chapter we will present some definitions of culture and, in particular, the concept of the hidden curriculum. We will talk about a key feature of the hidden curriculum: ingrained hierarchies and power asymmetries. We share four ways in which healthcare cultures (focusing on the hidden curriculum) can be revealed, using illustrative case studies from our own research programme (Monrouxe and Rees, 2017; see Further reading/resources). Finally, we end our chapter with a discussion of how healthcare cultures can be improved. We hope this chapter will help healthcare students, trainees and practitioners to navigate their way through complex healthcare cultures, and in doing so become agents of cultural change – not only to better protect themselves and their colleagues but also their patients.

What is culture?

Culture has been described as 'the total range of activities and ideas of a group of people with shared traditions, which are transmitted and reinforced by members of the group' (see http://www.collinsdictionary.com/dictionary/english/culture). Therefore, when we think of the healthcare culture, we largely consider the values and practices held by healthcare professionals that are simultaneously conveyed and bolstered by group members both explicitly and implicitly. From an educational perspective, the hidden curriculum commonly springs to mind when we contemplate healthcare culture, especially in relation to professionalism and professional

---

ABC of Clinical Professionalism, First Edition. Edited by Nicola Cooper, Anna Frain and John Frain.
© 2018 John Wiley & Sons Ltd. Published 2018 by John Wiley & Sons Ltd.

identity formation. Described variously in the literature (e.g., Hafferty, 1998; see Further reading/resources), the hidden curriculum has been defined as: 'elements of socialisation… not part of the formal curricular content. These include the norms, values, and belief systems embedded in the curriculum, the school, and classroom life, imparted to students through daily routines, curricular content, and social relationships' (Margolis, 2001; see Further reading/resources). It is essentially through the hidden curriculum that students receive oft-subtle yet powerful messages about what is and what is not valued within the institutional cultures in which they learn, including different healthcare settings, the medical school, and so on. Several research groups, including ourselves, have begun to document the 'content' of the hidden curriculum within medical education, with one of the key elements involving students learning about the multiplicity of healthcare hierarchies and their place within those hierarchies (Monrouxe and Rees, 2017; see Further reading/resources).

What about hierarchies and power in medicine?

Innumerable hierarchies exist in healthcare, with hierarchies relating to levels of training, specialities and healthcare professional groups. Irrespective of profession or speciality, those at higher levels of training are thought to assume more authority and power over junior staff. Across the different healthcare professions, doctors are often considered to be at the top of the healthcare hierarchies, while other professionals such as nurses are thought to be near the bottom (Monrouxe and Rees, 2017; see Further reading/resources). Furthermore, within medicine, prestige hierarchies are felt to exist within Western cultures with specialities with active, specialised, biomedical and technological characteristics such as surgery being afforded higher prestige than specialities with opposite qualities such as psychiatry [Norredam, M. and Album, D. (2007) Prestige and its significance for medical specialties and diseases. *Scandinavian Journal of Public Health*, **35**, 655–661]. This multiplicity of hierarchies imply power asymmetries between individuals at different levels of the hierarchies, with those at the top thought to be more powerful and those at the bottom powerless (Monrouxe and Rees, 2017; see Further reading/resources). However, we take a Foucauldian perspective on power in our research. Here, power is something that is continuously enacted and resisted through social interaction – by those in superordinate *and* subordinate positions – rather than something that is only wielded by those in positions of power and authority, such as consultants or consultant nurses (see Figure 6.1).

How do we experience medical culture?

Several authors have discussed how the hidden curriculum of learning organisations can be visibilised through examining, for example, the physical environment, the body, institutional slang including derogatory humour, and institutional policies [Gair, M. and Mullins, G. (2001) Hiding in Plain Sight, in E. Margolis (ed.), *The Hidden Curriculum in Higher Education*. Routledge, New York, pp. 21–41].

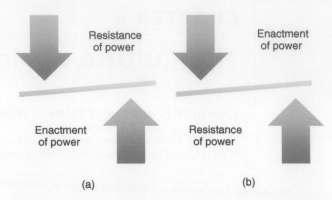

Figure 6.1 The enactment and resistance of power in workplace social interactions. This figure illustrates how those in ascribed superordinate and subordinate positions can both enact and resist power in workplace social interactions. For example, in (a) imagine the scenario of a clinical teacher enacting power with a student by failing the student's professionalism assessment, but the student resisting that power by formally complaining about his/her grade to the healthcare school. In (b), imagine the scenario of a patient enacting power with a student by physically threatening the student, but the student resisting that power by refusing to deliver care to the patient (Monrouxe, L.V. and Rees, C.E., 2017; see Further reading/ resources).

The physical environment

In terms of the physical environment, healthcare students can come to understand what is and what is not valued within the healthcare workplace through the buildings and the physical arrangement of clinical settings. For example, healthcare students in our study often talked about tensions between their professionalism teaching on the one hand, where the importance of maintaining patient dignity and privacy was stressed, and their live experiences of the physical hospital environment on the other hand, which often contravened patient dignity and privacy. This can be seen neatly in Gladys' narrative, a junior doctor from one of our studies, who explains how the flimsy curtains between beds on wards give only an illusion of patient privacy (see Box 6.1). Therefore, students can learn from the physical environment, as part of the hidden curriculum, that privacy is not as important as the formal curriculum might suggest.

The body

In terms of the body, scholars explain how the hidden curriculum is manifested in the gendered, racialised and class-based bodies of students and staff [Gair, M. and Mullins, G. (2001) Hiding in Plain

Box 6.1 **'The patient opposite was given a diagnosis of cancer behind the magic curtain.'**

"He [boyfriend] overheard a conversation with the patient opposite and the patient opposite was given, er, a diagnosis of, of, cancer behind the 'magic curtain' um, and [name] was quite upset that he'd heard this man's news. as had the rest of the bay potentially … I think that it's such a shame that so many difficult conversations, they might be had behind a curtain but it's because there isn't um the physical environment to make a more appropriate, have a conversation in a nicer setting."

Gladys, Junior Doctor, UK

Box 6.2 **'It's been a while since a young lady had a play with my balls.'**

"I was asked to perform a male genital examination by the GP. After obtaining consent [the] patient replied, '...sure, it's been a while since a young lady had a play with my balls'. [This took place in a GP surgery.] Present was myself, the senior GP, and [the] patient himself... [I did] nothing/ignored the comment. It was more tongue-in-cheek and [the] patient was probably nervous and said it to ease off tension. [I] feel mildly disturbed about the remark now. As a female student/soon [to be] junior doctor, this kind of incident seems to happen fairly often, especially with older male patients."

Simone, Female, Year 5, Medical Student, UK

Box 6.3 **'Both doctors started laughing over the joke.'**

"Two doctors [were] joking in front of a patient about the patient's impending leg amputation. I was a 3rd year med student on a vascular team. The Reg[istrar] and SHO [senior house officer] went to mark out the leg to be amputated on a patient... Doctor X commented saying '...seems silly but we need to make sure we get the right leg.' Doctor Y then goes "but you mean the left?" Both doctors started laughing over the joke. [The] patient looked like they were about to cry and [the] nurse went to comfort them. [I did] nothing. It was right in front of a patient and couldn't say anything there and then. It's been an uncommon occurrence, so feel it was a one off and that overall these two were good doctors."

John, Male, Year 5, Medical Student, UK

Sight, in E. Margolis (ed.), *The Hidden Curriculum in Higher Education*. Routledge, New York, pp. 21–41]. Healthcare students in our studies often talked about the physical manifestations of professionalism in terms of appearance, with students learning what constitutes a professional appearance through observing how healthcare professionals looked. Indeed, one of our male student participants explained that he equated a professional appearance with the doctor wearing a shirt, tie and a suit jacket, which conjures up a stereotypical image of *the* male doctor. Indeed, female medical students often alluded to medicine as a gendered environment (essentially male-dominated), and we can see this clearly though the numerous sexual harassment stories we collected from female medical students as part of our programme of professionalism research (Monrouxe and Rees, 2017; see Further reading/resources). As can be seen in Simone's narrative, she is learning through the hidden curriculum that medicine is male, and as a female medic she is to expect being on the receiving end of sexual innuendo and harassment from males in her professional workplace (see Box 6.2).

Institutional slang and derogatory humour

With respect to institutional slang, language is key in terms of communicating to healthcare students who is and is not valued within the healthcare workplace. This is no more important than the ways that healthcare practitioners refer to patients, including their use of derogatory descriptors such as 'mad', 'attention-seekers', 'time-wasters', and so on. This is keenly apparent in fictional books written by doctors, where patients may be referred to derogatorily as 'Gomers', meaning 'Get Out of My Emergency Room' [Shem, S. (1979) *The House of God*. Bodley Head, Great Britain]. While much has been written about doctors' use of institutional slang and derogatory humour, healthcare students can learn through such acts that it is acceptable (and even inevitable) that making fun of vulnerable patients is the best way of coping with their own emotional turmoil associated with medical work. This can be seen in John's narrative, where he witnesses two qualified doctors making jokes about a patient's leg amputation in front of the patient, causing the patient unnecessary distress ahead of their amputation. As we can see, John downplays these doctors' inappropriate humour as a one-off event in two otherwise 'good doctors', suggesting that he has already become inculcated into this practice (see Box 6.3).

Institutional policies

While the physical environment, staff and student bodies, institutional slang and derogatory humour are all non-intentional socialisation practices that help to visibilise the healthcare culture (or the hidden curriculum), we can also see the hidden curriculum through intentional socialisation practices such as via institutional policies. Indeed, one could argue that the formal professionalism curriculum itself (discussed later in Chapter 10) is an intentional socialisation practice to 'create' medical graduates with the 'right' values and habits of mind on graduation. Indeed, we found that healthcare students in our study were quite rule-bound in terms of their ways of conceptualising professionalism, particularly more junior healthcare students such as pre-clinical medical students. Such institutional policies and rule-following is apparent in Morgan's narrative (see Box 6.4), in which she recounts requesting supervision from her nurse mentor while she conducts an intramuscular injection on a patient. Interestingly, while Morgan appears to know what the institutional policy is and is keen to follow the rules, her nurse mentor's apparent disregard for the policy could communicate to Morgan that the supervision of students' procedural skills is not always necessary.

Box 6.4 **'I had to ask to be supervised as per clinical regulations/policy.'**

"I was asked whether I would like to give a patient an IM [intramuscular] injection by a qualified Mental Health Nurse [on a community mental health placement]... The nurse in question did not follow me into the room in which the injection would be given so as to supervise the procedure. With the patient present, I had to ask to be supervised as per clinical regulations/policy ... I know I am unable to undertake such a clinical procedure without the supervision of a relevant qualified professional present to observe.
I discussed/de-briefed the issue with my mentor and she informed me that I had not breached any policies/regulations as [she] did supervise me at my request. However, I felt that by me having to ask for the qualified member of staff to oversee the procedure in front of the patient... [this] may have been worrying for the patient and family."

Morgan, Female, Year 2, Nursing Student, UK

How can medical culture be improved?

In light of the inquiry into failings at the Mid Staffordshire NHS Foundation Trust in the UK, Francis (2013) recommended that 'a fundamental culture change is needed', and put forward 290 recommendations for changing the UK National Health Service culture (see Further reading/resources). Key recommendations at the individual level included the need for all individuals to provide safe and compassionate care, and at the organisational level included developing cultures of openness, transparency and candour and having zero tolerance for services not complying with the fundamental standards of care enshrined in the NHS constitution. In our previous research, we have argued that both strategies driven by leaders and those driven by healthcare students are needed to facilitate cultural change in the healthcare workplace.

In terms of strategies driven by students, while healthcare students and trainees are expected to raise their concerns about professionalism lapses, many feel unable to act in the face of such lapses; instead, going along with lapses because of their fears about the negative repercussions of challenging healthcare hierarchies (Rees *et al.*, 2013; see Further reading/resources). However, students who do act in the face of professionalism lapses typically choose strategies that are more indirect and subtle (and therefore lower risk), rather than choosing direct and blatant strategies of challenging the professionalism lapse perpetrators. This is clear in Tali's narrative, where she describes enacting various acts of resistance in the face of her consultant's perceived professionalism lapses (e.g., bodily acts of resistance, debriefing and reporting her perpetrator to her supervisor) rather than challenging the perpetrator directly (see Box 6.5). The most common types of resistance found in 680

> **Box 6.5 'I talked to the nurses… I then talked to the GP.'**
>
> *"I felt a consultant was conducting small operations in an unhygienic way and in an unsuitable room. I was in the general practice and only I and the O+G [obstetrics and gynaecologist] consultant and patient was in the room … I felt uncomfortable with the small operations she did as I felt this was not the correct room to be doing it in and the right situation (i.e., carpet on the floor). Also needles were put directly into the sink and in general hygiene levels [were] not high.* **I, at the time, didn't say anything to the consultant** *[no direct challenge of the perpetrator]*, **but I got antibacterial wipes to clean the areas (i.e., examination bench)** *[bodily act of resistance]*. **I also tried to get the needle and put it in the sharps bin quickly but safely** *[bodily act of resistance]*. **Later, I talked to the nurses who had worked with her before and they agreed with me about my opinions** *[debriefing with supportive people]*. **I then talked to the GP who was my supervisor and told him what had happened and my suggestions to change it** *[reported perpetrator to supervisor]. I felt I did not know the situation/protocol/individual enough to talk to the consultant, but I felt able to talk to others in the practice and make sure that the situation was brought to the forefront of their minds. I still feel that this was very bad practice and I hope that her clinic has been moved to the surgical room upstairs in the practice."*
>
> Tali, Female, Year 5, Medical Student, UK

UK medical students' written most-memorable lapses can be seen in Figure 6.2. We therefore encourage students who might be worried about direct challenges to instead enact indirect and more subtle resistance strategies in the face of professionalism lapses.

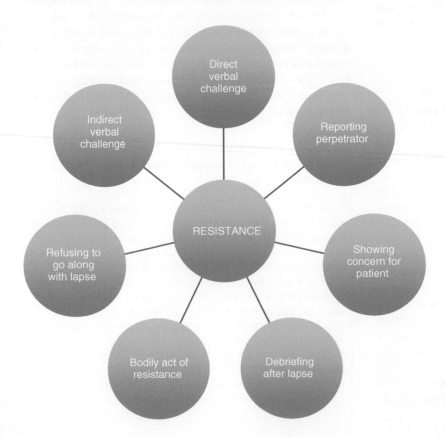

Figure 6.2 Common resistance strategies adopted by medical students in the face of professionalism lapses (C.E. Rees *et al.*, 2013; see Further reading/resources).

In terms of strategies driven by leaders, we know that the healthcare workplace often displays evidence of weak ethical cultures in which there is low agreement among members of those cultures about appropriate ethical behaviours and how ethical issues should be managed [Victor, B. and Cullen, J. (1987) A theory and measure of ethical climate in organization. *Research in Corporate Social Performance and Policy*, **9**, 51–71]. We know that institutional policies alone are inadequate in preventing professionalism lapses. Leaders instead need to develop and shape organisational values, to communicate those values through their role-modelling practices, as well as facilitating the good practices of others in positions of leadership. Leaders should also provide opportunities for learners and healthcare professionals to safely raise their concerns about suboptimal workplace practices, without fear of punishment or retribution.

Conclusions

This chapter has defined culture and the hidden curriculum and has provided insights into a key feature of the hidden curriculum, that is, ingrained hierarchies and power asymmetries. We have discussed four ways in which the healthcare culture (or hidden curriculum) can be visibilised – through the physical environment, bodies of staff and students, institutional slang and derogatory humour, and intentional socialisation practices – using illustrative case studies from our own research with healthcare students (Monrouxe and Rees, 2017; see Further reading/resources). Finally, we have concluded our chapter with a brief exploration of how the healthcare culture can be improved in the future, through attention to student- and leader-driven strategies. We hope that this chapter will help healthcare students, trainees and practitioners reflect critically on the healthcare culture and their place within it, alongside providing some encouragement to help them enact small cultural changes through acts of resistance which challenge the current status quo. We believe that such resistance is essential to improving the culture of healthcare, for the betterment of students, clinical teachers and patients.

Acknowledgements

This chapter is based on a decade-long research programme funded in parts by the British Academy, the Association for the Study of Medical Education, the Association for Medical Education in Europe, the Higher Education Academy, and NHS Education for Scotland. We thank the thousands of healthcare students who have participated in our professionalism research and shared their professionalism dilemmas with us so candidly. We also thank the numerous researchers who have worked with us to help collect and analyse professionalism data.

Further reading/resources

Francis, R. (2013) Report of the Mid Staffordshire NHS Foundation Trust Public Inquiry. Executive Summary. The Stationery Office, London.

Hafferty, F.W. (1998) Beyond curriculum reform: confronting medicine's hidden curriculum. *Academic Medicine*, **73** (4), 403–407.

Margolis, E. (2001) *The Hidden Curriculum in Higher Education*. Routledge, New York.

Monrouxe, L.V. and Rees, C.E. (2017) *Healthcare professionalism. Improving practice through reflections on workplace dilemmas*. Wiley-Blackwell, Oxford.

Rees, C.E., Monrouxe, L.V. and McDonald, L.A. (2013) Narrative, emotion, and action: Analysing 'most memorable' professionalism dilemmas. *Medical Education*, **47** (1), 80–96.

CHAPTER 7

Ensuring Patient Safety

Nicola Cooper

Derby Teaching Hospitals NHS Foundation Trust and Division of Graduate Entry Medicine, University of Nottingham, UK

OVERVIEW

- Healthcare professionals must 'first, do no harm'.

- However, preventable harm is common and costs the National Health Service (NHS) up to £2.5 billion each year.

- Errors are predictable and tend to repeat themselves in patterns, which is why incident reporting systems are so important.

- A just culture is one in which front-line operators and others are not punished for 'honest errors', but also where gross negligence, wilful violations and destructive acts are not tolerated.

- While the conditions in which we work sometimes make it difficult for us to act as we should, healthcare professionals have a duty to raise concerns about unsafe systems and processes, and follow standard operating procedures that are designed to keep patients safe.

Introduction

The UK General Medical Council's *Good Medical Practice* states that doctors must 'make the care of your patient your first concern' (see Box 7.1). This statement is a modern version of part of the ancient Hippocratic Oath in which physicians swore to 'first do no harm'. However, there is growing recognition that modern healthcare systems, and healthcare professionals who work in them, in fact do cause harm – although the rate of harm varies considerably in studies. A reasonable estimate would be to assume that in developed countries 10% of hospital in-patients are harmed by the healthcare system, and in 1% of cases this directly contributes to their deaths (see Further reading/resources).

The modern concept of patient safety is relatively new. It was born in the 1990s with publication of the Harvard Medical Practice Study (see Further reading/resources). The authors looked at sue-able adverse events in a small group of hospitals and calculated that, if the incidence was the same in all US hospitals, the harm caused was the equivalent of a fatal jumbo jet crash every day. It took several years before healthcare organisations and governments began to accept that significant avoidable harm

---

Box 7.1 General Medical Council: Good Medical Practice.

Patients must be able to trust doctors with their lives and health. To justify that trust you must show respect for human life and make sure your practice meets the standards expected of you in four domains:
- Knowledge, skills and performance:
  - Make the care of your patient your first concern.
  - Provide a good standard of practice and care – keep your professional knowledge and skills up to date. Recognise and work within the limits of your competence.
- Safety and quality:
  - Take prompt action if you think that patient safety, dignity or comfort is being compromised.
  - Protect and promote the health of patients and the public.
- Communication, partnership and teamwork:
  - Treat patients as individuals and respect their dignity.
  - Work in partnership with patients.
  - Work with colleagues in the ways that best serve patients' interests.
- Maintaining trust:
  - Be honest and open and act with integrity.
  - Never discriminate unfairly against patients or colleagues.
  - Never abuse your patients' trust in you or the public's trust in the profession.

You are personally accountable for your professional practice and must always be prepared to justify your decisions and actions.

From *Good Medical Practice*, 2013. http://www.gmc-uk.org/guidance/good_medical_practice/duties_of_a_doctor.asp (accessed October 2016).

---

was a problem. The landmark publication, *To Err is Human: Building a Safer Health System* (US Institute of Medicine, 1999) followed by the UK Government's *An Organisation with a Memory* (Department of Health, 2000) helped to kick-start the global patient safety movement that exists today.

It is clear that healthcare professionals have a duty to ensure patient safety. Many of us can think of behaviours we need to adopt to protect individual patients (e.g., washing our hands with soap

---

ABC of Clinical Professionalism, First Edition. Edited by Nicola Cooper, Anna Frain and John Frain.
© 2018 John Wiley & Sons Ltd. Published 2018 by John Wiley & Sons Ltd.

and water after seeing a patient with diarrhoea and vomiting). However, the bigger picture is just as important. Healthcare professionals need to understand the science of patient safety and their responsibilities as part of a team, as part of a 'complex system', and a wider healthcare organisation, as this chapter will illustrate.

What is 'patient safety'?

The World Health Organization defines patient safety this way: 'The simplest definition of patient safety is the prevention of errors and adverse events to patients associated with healthcare. While healthcare has become more effective it has also become more complex, with greater use of new technologies, medicines and treatments'.

Errors and adverse events are not the same thing. An *error* is an unintended act (either of omission or commission) or one that does not achieve its intended outcome. This could be due to the failure of a planned action to be completed as intended (an error of execution), the use of a wrong plan to achieve an aim (an error of planning), or a deviation from the process of care. An *adverse event* is what happens when an error results in harm to a patient. Patient harm can occur at an individual or system level.

Errors are inevitable in a complex system such as healthcare. Even if a 600-bed hospital managed to eliminate errors by 99.9%, there would still be 4000 drug errors each year. The most important thing we need to understand about errors is that, to an extent, *they are predictable and tend to repeat themselves in patterns*. The system in which we work can either adapt for this and make errors (and resulting adverse events) less likely, or it can in fact create 'accidents waiting to happen'. Pause for a minute to consider your own workplace.

Errors are unlikely to go reported when the patient has not come to any harm. In the 1930s it was estimated that for every one major injury there were 29 minor injuries and 300 'no harm' accidents (Heinrich's Law; see Figure 7.1). Because many accidents share

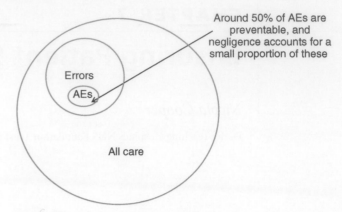

Figure 7.2 Error, adverse events, preventable adverse events and negligence. AEs = adverse events.

common root causes, addressing the causes of more commonplace incidents that cause no injuries can prevent accidents that cause serious injuries. While things have certainly changed since that time, the idea that adverse events are just the 'tip of the iceberg' has not changed. This is the reason why anonymous incident reporting is mandatory in the aviation industry and has contributed to a better understanding of how systems can be improved to make errors and adverse events less likely.

Not all adverse events are preventable. For example, if a patient with no known allergies suffers an allergic reaction to penicillin, that is an adverse event that could not have been prevented. But if a patient with a known allergy to penicillin is given a penicillin by accident and comes to harm, that *is* a preventable adverse event. Studies vary, but at least half of adverse events are considered to be preventable.

Research commissioned by the Department of Health estimated that preventable adverse events cost the NHS up to £2.5 billion each year, or 2.5% of England's NHS budget.

Figure 7.2 illustrates the relationship between error, adverse events, preventable adverse events and negligence.

Understanding why things go wrong

Understanding the scale of error in healthcare is important, but so is understanding the nature of error. If it is our professional duty to make the care of the patient our first concern, and to work with colleagues in the ways that best serve patients' interests (see Box 7.1) then understanding *why* things go wrong is vital in order to prevent harm.

Serious adverse events tend to occur after a series of smaller things go wrong. This is referred to as an 'error chain' and has been famously described in the 'Swiss Cheese model of accident causation' (see Fig 7.3). If we imagine blood transfusion as a common example, it has a series of defences, barriers and safeguards in place to prevent harm to patients – from selection of donors, to screening and treatment of blood products, labelling, storage, ordering and finally administering. If any of these procedures are faulty, or are not strictly followed – that is, if there are holes – then on any given day these could align and cause a fatal patient safety incident.

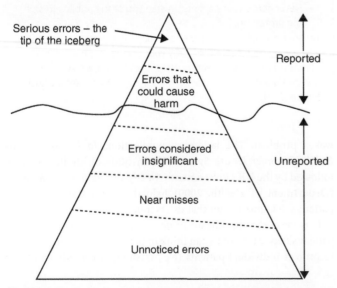

Figure 7.1 Heinrich's Law. Reproduced with permission from Cooper, N. (2006) Why things go wrong, in *Essential Guide to Generic Skills* (eds N. Cooper, K. Forrest and P. Cramp), Wiley-Blackwell.

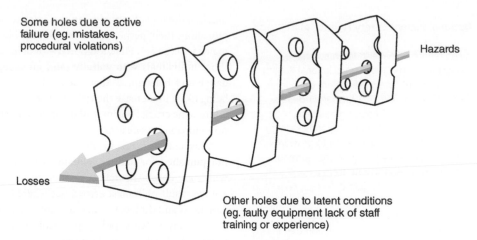

Some holes due to active failure (eg. mistakes, procedural violations)

Hazards

Losses

Other holes due to latent conditions (eg. faulty equipment lack of staff training or experience)

Successive layers of defences, barriers and safeguards

Figure 7.3 The Swiss Cheese model of accident causation. Reproduced with permission from Reason, J. (1991) *Human Error*. Cambridge University Press.

This understanding of the nature of serious incidents has led to the concept of 'root cause analysis' in healthcare. There are frequently problems with systems and processes that make an accident likely to happen, as well as 'human factors' (see Box 7.2). Blaming an individual when something goes wrong is an inaccurate and damaging perspective, and more importantly does nothing to prevent the same thing from happening again.

As healthcare professionals, this understanding of error and harm helps us to understand why we have a duty to raise concerns about unsafe systems and processes, follow standard operating procedures that are designed to keep patients safe, and report incidents including near misses using our organisation's incident reporting system. A good understanding of error and harm also helps us to support colleagues who commit errors or who are involved in patient safety incidents.

Reporting and learning systems

Incident reporting is the main way an organisation can learn and implement changes in its systems and processes to make them safer. In high-risk industries, such as aviation, incident reporting is well developed. These industries focus on safety, anticipate adverse events, and encourage incident and near-miss reporting. If healthcare is to become safer, we need to do the same. The following is a list of examples of incidents that should be reported routinely, including near misses:

- Medication errors.
- Adverse drug reactions.
- Equipment faults or equipment not available.
- Patient injury as a result of a procedure (which may be a recognised complication).
- Care not as intended.
- Patient care adversely affected for non-clinical reasons (e.g., no ICU bed available).
- Injuries (including falls and needle stick injuries).

For incidents with serious consequences, for example, death or serious injury, there is a separate 'serious untoward incident' process. The UK also has a National Reporting and Learning System (NRLS) that receives patient safety incident reports from local databases. This data is then analysed to identify hazards, risks and opportunities to improve safety. The system is the most comprehensive of its kind in the world, and since it was established in 2003 it has received over four million incident reports. The National Patient Safety Agency uses this information to issue national patient safety alerts (see Box 7.3).

Since 2014, NHS professionals have had a legal duty of candour which means informing patients or their relatives about any incident, providing reasonable support, providing truthful information and an apology. The NHS Litigation Authority has produced guidance on the importance of saying sorry: 'Saying sorry when things go wrong is vital for the patient, their family and carers, as well as to support learning and improve safety. Of those that have suffered harm as a result of their healthcare, fifty percent wanted an apology and explanation. Patients, their families and carers should receive a meaningful apology – one that is a sincere expression of sorrow or regret for the harm that has occurred'. The guidance goes on to explain that poor communication makes it more likely that people will pursue a formal complaint or claim. 'Saying sorry is not an admission of liability; it is the right thing to do'.

Box 7.2 Human factors.

Human factors is the science of the limitations of human performance. Increasingly, healthcare professionals are being trained in human factors and this training covers:

- The patterns and causes of error.
- The limitations of human performance.
- Situation awareness and team communication.

Analysis of serious adverse events in clinical practice shows that human factors – and poor team communication in particular – play a significant role when things go wrong. Examples of the limitations of human performance are seen when things like poor equipment design, fatigue, interruptions and excessive workload make accidents more likely to occur.

'In February 2005, following reports of patient death and harm caused by misplaced nasogastric feeding tubes, the National Patient Safety Agency (NPSA) issued a Patient Safety Alert. Between September 2005 and March 2010 there were a further 21 deaths and 79 cases of harm, related to feeding through misplaced nasogastric tubes, reported to the National Reporting and Learning System. We have therefore updated our original Alert to provide organisations with strengthened guidance based on the learning from these reports. In 2009 feeding into the lung from a misplaced nasogastric tube became a Never Event in England'.

March 2011

http://www.nrls.npsa.nhs.uk/alerts (accessed October 2016).

The NPSA issued guidance on equipment and a decision tree for clinical staff to follow to ensure that nasogastric tubes were safe to use. All healthcare organisations are expected to follow this guidance.

Just culture versus blame culture

Safety experts emphasise the importance of a 'just culture', and all healthcare professionals have a duty to nurture this. James Reason, psychologist and expert in human error, wrote that (see Further reading/resources), "The term 'no-blame' culture flourished in the 1990s and still endures today. Compared to the largely punitive cultures it sought to replace, it was clearly a step in the right direction. It acknowledged that a large proportion of unsafe acts were 'honest errors' (the kinds of slips, lapses and mistakes that even the best people can make) and were not truly blameworthy, nor was there

much in the way of remedial or preventative benefit to be had from punishing their perpetrators. But the 'no-blame' concept had two major weaknesses. First, it ignored – or at least, failed to confront – those individuals who wilfully (and often repeatedly) engaged in dangerous behaviours that most observers would recognise as being likely to increase the risk of a bad outcome. Second, it did not address the crucial business of distinguishing between culpable and non-culpable unsafe acts".

A just culture is one in which front-line operators and others are not punished for actions, omissions or decisions taken by them which are commensurate with their experience and training and are the result of 'honest errors', but where gross negligence, wilful violations and destructive acts are not tolerated.

With any process, policy, protocol or regulation in healthcare there is the legal/expected safe space of action – the way things are supposed to be done. But there is frequently pressure, or demand that pushes us to take shortcuts and do things a little differently, occasionally for good clinical reasons. Normally, migration from standard procedures is limited to 'borderline tolerated conditions' (the 'illegal–normal' space in Figure 7.4). Staff tacitly accept routine minor violations, while weighing the risks.

Violations and migration from standard procedure occurs frequently in life and in all industries, even those with very good safety records. Violations are a complex phenomenon – they occur frequently and may save time and bring benefits. They may be tolerated and even encouraged if there is pressure to increase the throughput of patients, for example. Incident reporting systems are poor at detecting them.

However, depending on the organisational culture, staffing levels and attitudes to safety, violations may become so routine and

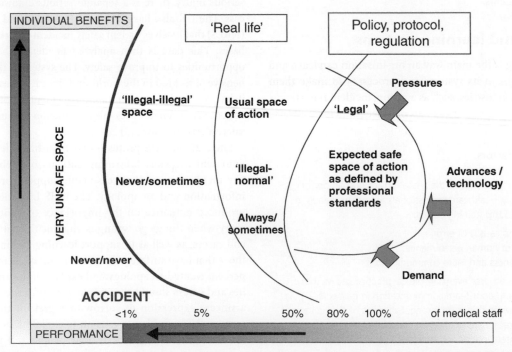

Figure 7.4 Systemic migration to boundaries. Adapted from Amalberti, R., Vincent, C., Auroy, Y. and Saint Maurice, G. (2006) Violations and migrations in healthcare: a framework for understanding and management. *Quality and Safety in Healthcare*, **15**, 66–71.

normalised as to become invisible. This 'normalisation of deviance' can result in patient harm when a small number of individuals are willing to violate basic procedures to the point of recklessness. It could be argued that this was what was going on in the now well-known Mid Staffordshire NHS Foundation Trust inquiry in which patients were harmed through neglect.

In terms of professionalism, what does this mean?

Professionalism and patient safety

The 2005 Royal College of Physicians of London report, *Doctors in Society: Medical Professionalism in a Changing World*, stated that 'The exercise of medical professionalism is hampered by the political and cultural environment of health, which many doctors consider disabling'. In other words, sometimes the conditions in which we work can make it difficult to act as we would like. However, the report goes on to state, 'Professionalism therefore implies multiple commitments – to the patient, to fellow professionals, and to the institution or system in which healthcare is provided, to the extent that the system supports patients collectively. A doctor's corporate responsibility, shared as it is with managers and others, is a frequently neglected aspect of modern practice'.

Doctors, and all healthcare professionals, have a responsibility to work with others to create safe organisations and processes of care and to speak up if this is not the case, even if that is difficult (see Box 7.4). The Royal College of Physicians definition of medical professionalism is shown in Box 7.5.

Conclusions

As we have seen, ensuring patient safety is not only about a person's individual behaviour, although that is important. It is also about

---

> Box 7.5 **Royal College of Physicians' definition of professionalism.**
>
> 'Medical professionalism signifies a set of values, behaviours and relationships that underpins the trust the public has in doctors.
>
> Medicine is a vocation in which a doctor's knowledge, clinical skills and judgement are put in the service of protecting and restoring human well-being. This purpose is realised through a partnership between patient and doctor, one based on mutual respect, individual responsibility, and appropriate accountability.
>
> In their day-to-day practice, doctors are committed to:
>
> - Integrity.
> - Compassion.
> - Altruism.
> - Continuous improvement.
> - Excellence.
> - Working in partnership with members of the wider healthcare team.
>
> These values, which underpin the science and practice of medicine, form the basis for a moral contract between the medical profession and society. Each party has a duty to work to strengthen the system of healthcare on which our collective human dignity depends.'
>
> From Royal College of Physicians of London. *Doctors in Society: Medical Professionalism in a Changing World*. Report of a working party. RCP, December 2005. http://shop.rcplondon.ac.uk/products/doctors-in-society-medical-professionalism-in-a-changing-world?variant=6337443013 (accessed October 2016).

---

our role in the wider healthcare team and the systems and organisations in which we work.

As an individual we have a professional responsibility to understand what patient safety is and the science behind it. 'Boring' adherence to organisational policies, whether it be correct aseptic no-touch technique when inserting a cannula, team briefings before theatre lists, participating in safety huddles, incident reporting, mandatory training or following correct protocols for medical procedures – these are important for patient safety. If you see a way in which things could be improved, work with others to improve things. If you see a pattern of repeating errors, work with others to change the process to make it easier for people to do the right thing. If you are not in a position to do this, talk to someone who is. Gain a basic understanding of patient safety and quality improvement methods. But above all, think in terms of teams, processes and systems as well as yourself – because it is these that ultimately look after patients in modern healthcare systems, not individuals.

> Box 7.4 **General Medical Council: Good Medical Practice. Domain 2 – Quality and Safety.**
>
> **Respond to risks to safety**
>
> You must promote and encourage a culture that allows all staff to raise concerns openly and safely.
>
> You must take prompt action if you think that patient safety, dignity or comfort is or may be seriously compromised.
>
> **a** If a patient is not receiving basic care to meet their needs, you must immediately tell someone who is in a position to act straight away.
>
> **b** If patients are at risk because of inadequate premises, equipment or other resources, policies or systems, you should put the matter right if that is possible. You must raise your concern in line with our guidance and your workplace policy. You should also make a record of the steps you have taken.
>
> **c** If you have concerns that a colleague may not be fit to practise and may be putting patients at risk, you must ask for advice from a colleague, your defence body, or us. If you are still concerned you must report this, in line with our guidance and your workplace policy, and make a record of the steps you have taken.
>
> From *Good Medical Practice*, 2013. http://www.gmc-uk.org/guidance/good_medical_practice/duties_of_a_doctor.asp (accessed October 2016).

Further reading/resources

Vincent, C., Neale, G. and Woloshynowych, M. (2001) Adverse events in British hospitals: a preliminary retrospective record review. *British Medical Journal*, **322**, 517–519.

Brennan, T.A., Leape, L.L., Laird, N.M. *et al.* (1991) Incidence of adverse events and negligence in hospitalised patients. *New England Journal of Medicine*, **324**, 370–376 [Harvard Medical Practice Study].

Department of Health (2000) An organisation with a memory. Report of an expert group on learning from adverse events in the NHS. Department of Health, London. http://patientsafety.health.org.uk/resources/organisation-memory (accessed October 2016).

Vincent, C. (2005) *Patient Safety*. Churchill-Livingstone, London.

Global Aviation Information Network (2004) A roadmap to a just culture: enhancing the safety environment. GAIN. www.flightsafety.org/files/just_culture.pdf (accessed October 2016).

Royal College of Physicians of London (2005) *Doctors in Society: Medical Professionalism in a Changing World*. Report of a working party. Royal College of Physicians. http://shop.rcplondon.ac.uk/products/doctors-in-society-medical-professionalism-in-a-changing-world?variant=6337443013 (accessed October 2016).

CHAPTER 8

Leadership and Collaboration

Judy McKimm[1] and Jill Thistlethwaite[2]

[1] Swansea University Medical School, Swansea University, UK
[2] University of Technology Sydney and School of Education, University of Queensland, Australia

OVERVIEW

- Contemporary health services require practitioners and organisations to work collaboratively for optimum patient-centred care.
- Collaboration and teamwork demand leadership, management and followership skills.
- Effective leadership provides motivation, direction and clarity on team goals, roles, processes and outcomes.
- Adaptive, inclusive and collective leadership approaches are best suited to collaborative practice.
- Communication and relationship building are central to successful collaborations.

Table 8.1 Leadership approaches and collaborative practice.

Leadership approach	Key features in terms of collaborative practice
Adaptive leadership	• Facilitates people to wrestle with the adaptive challenges for which there is no obvious solution – 'wicked problems'.
Complex leadership	• Comfortable to work in complex, ambiguous, uncertain worlds.
Collaborative, collective, shared leadership	• A mind-set that wants all those affected to be included and consulted. • Working together (through networks, partnerships) to identify and achieve shared goals. • The more power we share, the more power we have.
Distributed, dispersed leadership	• Involve informal, social process within organizations. • Open boundaries, expertise can lie anywhere in the organization. • Leadership is at all levels, leadership is everyone's responsibility.
Inclusive leadership	• Welcomes diversity, surfaces unconscious bias. • Strength is in diversity of views, ideas, expertise and experience.
Person-centred leadership	• Centred on knowing and sharing why you do what you do. Encouraging others regularly and intentionally, operating from your strengths and allowing others to compensate for your weaknesses (reflects person-centred care).
Servant, value-led, moral leadership	• Leader serves to serve first, then aspires to lead. • Concept of stewardship is important. • Values and morals underpin approaches and behaviours.
Transformational leadership	• Leads through transforming others to reach higher order goals or vision. • Role modelling, motivating, inspiring and attending to individuals is central. • Used widely in public services.

Introduction

Leadership is a key professional attribute. Being able to step up when leadership is required is essential for good patient care, and a lack of (or poor) leadership has a very damaging effect on individuals, teams and organisations. In contemporary health services, leaders from different organisations and professions need to work collaboratively so that the best healthcare can be provided to individuals and communities. Some leadership approaches are, however, more appropriate and effective than others in such dynamic, fluid contexts, and it is these we focus on in this chapter (see Table 8.1).

Working collaboratively

There are a number of definitions of collaboration (Box 8.1), but the word at its simplest means 'working together'. While collaboration encompasses teamwork, it also refers to less formal interactions with colleagues from one's own profession, to other health and social care professionals, managers and support workers working together to deliver effective and safe patient care. Collaboration can also be more formal, in terms of partnerships or other agreements between departments or organisations. Examples of collaborative practice are given in Box 8.2.

In most countries, health services are provided by a workforce including practitioners and support staff with diverse roles and responsibilities. The majority of patients in their lifetimes come into contact with many different health professionals both through inter- and intra-professional referrals, as well as self-referrals such

ABC of Clinical Professionalism, First Edition. Edited by Nicola Cooper, Anna Frain and John Frain.
© 2018 John Wiley & Sons Ltd. Published 2018 by John Wiley & Sons Ltd.

as to emergency departments. In order for care to be optimal, it is important that everyone involved with a particular patient or family communicates effectively, discussing diagnoses, prognoses and management plans, with the patient fully involved in decisions. Multi-disciplinary, multi-professional or inter-professional teams, whilst having differences in approach (Figure 8.1), are formally constructed and should meet regularly to plan and review goals and performance. Looser collaborations require other means of communication to ensure continuity and reduce fragmented care. Whatever the form of the collaboration, leadership is required to set direction and check that goals are being achieved in accordance with different stakeholders' needs and expectations. Leadership is only one element in a skill set that supports effective collaboration however; practitioners also need to be able to follow others appropriately and manage the processes and procedures that underpin collaboration. Figure 8.2 sets out the three elements of the 'leadership triad': leadership, management and followership. Each of these elements has a different set of activities associated with it, but all must interact smoothly to ensure that the collaboration works well. The case study in Box 8.3 shows how leadership is dispersed and shared across professional and hierarchical boundaries, the need for good management of the process to meet deadlines, and a collaborative, inclusive leadership approach in which leaders and followers work together to achieve aims.

All health professionals need an understanding of other professionals' roles, responsibilities, values, scope of practice, autonomy and reporting lines. This helps reduce misunderstandings and conflicting messages. Collaborative practice is a skill that needs to be learned, with appropriate knowledge of and respect for one's colleagues. It may sometimes involve conflict, and therefore negotiation, even when everyone involved is taking a patient- (or client- or family-) centred approach. While the medical doctor may frequently be the clinical leader of a team, with more integrated and dispersed service delivery, this is not inevitable.

If we add the adjective 'inter-professional' as a prefix to collaborative practice, we should expect high-quality care delivery, with

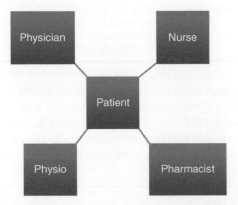

Multi-professional: each profession interacts with the patient but not with each other

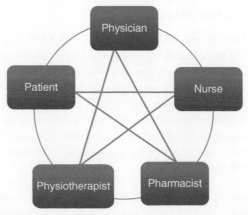

Interprofessional: each professional and the patient communicate with each other

Figure 8.1 Multi-professional and inter-professional collaboration.

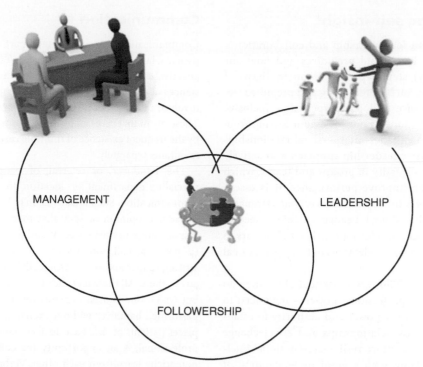

Figure 8.2 The 'leadership triad'.

Box 8.3 Case study: The 'leadership triad' in practice.

Ahmed, a doctor in training, has been asked by his consultant to work on a large quality improvement project to review and streamline maternity services in the hospital where he is working. He is asked to lead on carrying out the review in a fairly short timeframe. His consultant has some ideas about the changes that should be made, but she wants to devolve leadership so as to gain a wider range of views before presenting this to the board. Aware that this will have a huge impact on patients and staff, and not wanting to offend or miss anyone out of the review, Ahmed recognises he is not the 'expert' and will need help. He seeks the advice of one of the senior midwives in the department who he gets on well with and respects. She tells him that the new head of department has just completed a PhD which looked at international models of design for midwifery services. Ahmed goes to see the head to ask for her help in the review and specifically in pulling together a team who can collaborate on this task. Together they make a project plan with key activities identified so that he meets his deadline; she offers to identify key stakeholders and provides one of the administrator's help to send out invitations, plan a series of meetings and type up the notes. The review is completed on time with wide involvement and agreement. And whilst the recommendations are very different from the ones the consultant had originally envisaged, she is pleased how well Ahmed and the team have collaborated to provide the evidence for service improvement.

the different professionals providing health and social care through coordination and planning to meet what may well be disparate needs of patients. Ideally, the results are an individualised care plan,

which may be difficult to achieve but which does maximise the value of shared expertise.

Leading collaboratively

Leading collaboratively requires a shift in thinking from the traditional 'command and control' or 'heroic', individually oriented leadership style to one that is more flexible, adaptive and can work across professional and organisational boundaries (Table 8.1). A number of terms reflect this approach, including collaborative, shared, distributed and collective leadership. What these approaches have in common is:

- A mind-set that genuinely wants to work in collaboration, and can see the benefits for patients and communities.
- A focus on establishing a culture of collaboration, with shared responsibility for actions.
- A view of leadership that is vested in teams and groups, not individual leaders.
- That while leadership might reflect position or role, leaders can and should disperse leadership through organisations or teams.
- A willingness to share (even give away) power.
- A recognition that everyone can take on leadership roles and should be empowered to do so as appropriate.

This way of conceptualising leadership also recognises the importance of 'followers' to effective collaboration. The relationship between leaders and their followers is dynamic and fluid – it is not a one-way process where the leader commands and followers blindly obey. Followers have a lot of power in the way they moderate leaders' behaviours and how they define and create leaders. It therefore important to learn when and how to follow a 'good' leader, and to be able to challenge poor leadership appropriately.

Self-awareness and self-insight

Self-awareness is important for leadership and collaboration – understanding one's own biases and prejudices and how one may (often unconsciously) stereotype people on the basis of age, gender and profession. Such stereotyping and prejudice frequently arise from ignorance and past experience. Inclusive leaders will challenge and address poor behaviour arising from these attitudes in order to enhance interpersonal relationships and patient care. An inclusive leadership approach also actively and proactively welcomes diversity in groups and teams, which strengthens teams and can improve performance. It is essential to be able to work in a way that optimises everyone's strengths to achieve an identified shared goal. Leaders therefore need to actually hold these values and model appropriate behaviours in their day-to-day working: these are elements of transformational leadership.

Collaborative leaders and followers – particularly if they do not have high positional or professional power – may need to draw on their personal qualities, power and authority to establish credibility, build effective relationships and effect change (see Box 8.4). This takes time, effort, resilience, emotional intelligence and emotional labour, with a good understanding of one's strengths, weaknesses and impact on others. Developing self-insight and practical wisdom ('phronesis') can be achieved through purposeful, honest reflection, feedback from trusted colleagues or peers, and other development opportunities, such as unconscious bias, assertiveness or communication skills training.

Box 8.4 Personal skills required for effective collaboration. Reproduced from ABC of Clinical Leadership, 1st edition by Tim Swanwick .

- Building trust and credibility.
- Finding the common ground and defining a mutual intent to inspire action.
- Asking questions and seeking examples that illustrate what is meant.
- Emotional intelligence, active listening and 'walking in the shoes' of your collaborator.
- Advocating your point of view without harming your collaborator's feelings.
- Being clear, avoiding ambiguity and duplication of effort.
- Spotting when a conversation gets emotional, then making it safe again to continue meaningful dialogue.
- Telling and eliciting stories, conversation and dialogue.
- Being able to get things done, so you have something to show ('visible wins').
- Networking, being a 'connector' across people and systems.
- Showing that you are willing to learn and don't know everything.
- Acknowledging others' expertise, experience and knowledge.
- Being able to live with outcomes that may not be what you anticipated as long as they improve patient care or outcomes.
- Being resilient and able to handle conflict.
- Showing humility and being able to apologise.

Communication

Communication is an important part of collaboration. As with patients, language barriers due to professional jargon may impede effective communication. Details of the biopsychosocial circumstances of patients are frequently distributed between professionals involved in care, with no one person having complete information. These mean that care can become fragmented, a problem worsened by the frequent existence of multiple case notes that each profession maintains separately.

The 'handover', or referral, of patient care from one team, speciality, department or location to another requires optimal communication. Such a transfer may be permanent or temporary, for advice, opinion or specialist management. The process shifts responsibility to the new team and may be carried out face-to-face (if potential collaborators are co-located), on the telephone, in writing (paper and/or electronically) or through a combination of any of these. All these methods have advantages and disadvantages, but which one is used depends on the particular context. Poorly performed handover without exchange of significant information places patients at risk. Face-to-face handover, particularly if interprofessional, is an opportunity for collaborators to interact and potentially learn from each other. Verbal interaction should however be combined with written instructions.

Teamwork

'Team' is another word with a variety of meanings, depending on the context; however, all teams need certain factors to be in place to support collaboration (see Box 8.5). The influential US organisation, the Institute of Medicine (2001), has designated effective teamwork as a means of dealing with the increasing complexity of, and technological advances in, diagnosis and healthcare delivery. In healthcare, 'teams' may change membership frequently, such as when students and doctors in training move onto new rotations, while some remain constant over many years, for example primary care teams within general practices. Many health workers work in multiple teams and must learn to build good working relationships quickly with numerous people. 'Teams' also form for specific tasks, such as dealing with a cardiac arrest – for such events the health professionals should know their defined roles, even if they have not worked together before.

Box 8.5 Important factors for collaborative practice.

- Mutual performance monitoring: 'The ability to develop common understandings of the team environment and apply appropriate task strategies to accurately monitor teammate performance' (Salas *et al.*, 2005, p. 560).
- Psychological safety: a shared belief that the team is safe for interpersonal risk-taking; team members feel accepted and respected.
- Shared mental models: shared understanding of the task that is to be performed and of the involved teamwork.
- Structured handover: templates for communication ensure that all relevant information is included, for example ISBAR (identify, situation, background, assessment and recommendation).

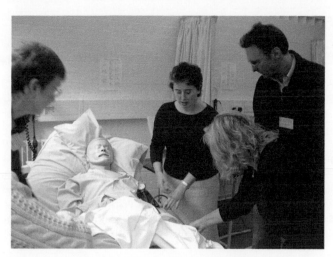

Figure 8.3 Team-based simulation can help teams work together more effectively. Reproduced with permission from Nicola Cooper.

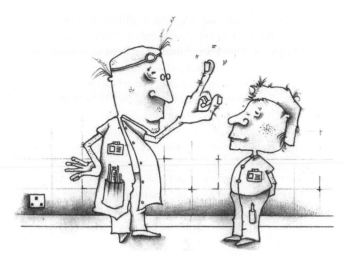

Figure 8.4 Toxic leaders do not reward or praise people; set unrealistic deadlines and expectations; and display passive-aggressive behaviours. Reproduced with permission from Cooper, N., Forrest, K. and Cramp, P. (2006) How to give feedback, in *Essential Guide to Generic Skills*. Blackwell-BMJ, Oxford.

Team leaders need to ensure that they keep both tasks and group processes in mind. Effective teams have clear, defined leadership, although (as in the cardiac arrest example above) the leadership might shift over time, depending on context and the expertise and role of those involved. Clear communication at all times helps to clarify the leader's role. A well-functioning team displays almost seamless 'handover' between leaders and followers as people step up and step back to carry out various activities. Team-based simulation can help teams work together more effectively through observation, debriefing, feedback, discussion and reflection (Figure 8.3).

While most people have worked or played in some form of team before entering higher education, they may not have had any formal teaching about teamwork or the health service in which they will eventually practise. Many health professional programmes now include learning outcomes related to teamwork and collaborative practice as part of inter-professional education (IPE) initiatives. Evidence shows, however, that students rarely feel they are part of a team. This is partly because they are moved frequently during their programmes in order to experience a range of clinical placements and locations. A notable way of enhancing 'belonging', which helps to improve understanding of how teams function, is the longitudinal integrated clinical placement (LIC), during which students are attached to one team with one supervisor in one location for more than 13 weeks, sometimes even for one year.

Dysfunctional collaboration

Collaboration and teamwork become dysfunctional for several reasons, which have implications for professionalism. Leadership is important, but an individual leader's style or approach and the choice of leader may not be acceptable to all. Personal or professional disagreements may affect morale and team spirit. Members may take sides. Power differentials and hierarchies may be problematic. More inexperienced staff can find it difficult to challenge senior professionals, while bullying can occur in any workplace. When health professionals are promoted, they may

not receive adequate and appropriate training in leadership or 'people' management.

Poor working relationships stem from and lead to poor trust in colleagues, avoidance of conflict, burnout, lack of motivation and commitment, and loss of accountability. Destructive or 'toxic' leaders typically undermine people; engage in malicious gossip; do not reward or praise people; set unrealistic deadlines and expectations; do not pull their weight; display passive-aggressive behaviours, and break promises (Figure 8.4). 'Pacesetting' or 'task focused' leadership can also be ineffective in collaborative teams, as time needs to be taken to bring people on board and build relationships – attention to group processes and dynamics is therefore vital. Destructive leadership behaviours need to be challenged but, depending on the team dynamics and internal power structures, this may be carried out more optimally by someone from outside the team. Dysfunctional teams may be helped by team meetings and team-building activities, again, sometimes with outside consultants, to diagnose difficulties and facilitate better working relationships. However, such remediation is more challenging in workplaces for people who do not work in the same team, as often no mechanisms exist to deal with these interrelationships.

Collaboration, change and complexity

Collaboration not only happens between and within teams, but also at organisational and system level. Such collaborations are more likely to rest on formal partnerships, networks, coalitions or alliances, established to effect service change or health improvements. Effecting larger-scale change requires an understanding of complex adaptive systems – systems that have properties over and above their component structures. In collaborative change projects, more than one system or many organisations (e.g., hospitals, community healthcare providers, social care providers) might be involved. This multiplies the complexity of the task and relationships involved and requires a different approach from managing a more linear type of change project, such as moving offices. Leaders of complex collaborations need to display 'adaptive leadership' – awareness of and willingness to work with ambiguities, uncertainties and dynamic and fluid relationships. They need to be aware of the possible impact of factors in both the external and internal environments, and may not necessarily have all the answers. Their role is to move the change initiative towards implementation through building consensus and agreement, and providing enough stability and certainty about what the change will involve and its impact on stakeholders, so that those involved remain empowered, engaged and motivated. Through such purposeful collaboration, large-scale, system change can emerge which can potentially be transformational.

Further reading/resources

Canadian Interprofessional Health Collaborative (2010) *A National Interprofessional Competency Framework*. 2010. http://www.cihc.ca/files/CIHC_IPCompetenciesShort_Feb1210.pdf (accessed 3 July 2016).

Dawson, J.F., Yan, X. and West, M.A. (2007) *Positive and negative effects of team working in healthcare: Real and pseudo-teams and their impact on safety*. Report, Aston University, Birmingham.

Hammick, M., Freeth, D., Copperman, J. and Goodsman, D. (2009) *Being Interprofessional*. Polity, Cambridge.

Institute of Medicine (2001) *Crossing the Quality Chasm: A new health system for the 21st century*. National Academy Press, Washington, DC.

Johnson, D.W. and Johnson, F.P. (2006) Group dynamics, in *Joining Together: Group Theory and Group Skills*. 9th edition. Pearson International, USA.

Salas, E., Sims, D.E. and Shawn Burke, C. (2005) Is there a 'big five' in teamwork? *Small Group Research*, **36**, 555–599. DOI: 10.1177/1046496405277134

CHAPTER 9

Ethical and Legal Aspects of Professionalism

Andrew Papanikitas

Nuffield Department of Primary Care Health Sciences, University of Oxford, UK

OVERVIEW

- Healthcare professionals need ways of understanding professional duties and reconciling them when they conflict.

- Being aware of the competing philosophies in western healthcare may help professionals practice with integrity and be better aware of conflicts.

- The Law defines what professionals may or may not do, but this requires further interpretation when applied to practice.

- Professional boundaries include understanding the clinician's power in a therapeutic relationship, but also the purpose of care, personal limitations and competence.

- Inter-professional working in healthcare means understanding that different professionals may have different ethical priorities, be trained for different aspects of practice, and be under different competing pressures.

- Probity and integrity are about how a professional upholds the right ethical values, and is as relevant to clinical care as it is to financial transactions or honesty in examinations and job interviews.

Box 9.1 **Six domains of medical professionalism.**

Personal (intrinsic) attributes of professionals:
1. Ethical practice.
2. Reflection and self-awareness.
3. Responsibility/accountability for actions (commitment to excellence/lifelong learning/critical reasoning).

Cooperative attributes of professionals:
4. Respect for patients.
5. Working with others (teamwork).
6. Social responsibility.

Adapted from Hilton, S. and Slotnick, H. (2005) Proto-professionalism: how professionalisation occurs across the continuum of medical education. *Medical Education*, **39** (1), 58–65.

Introduction

Most definitions of healthcare professionalism will include some definition of doing good, avoiding harm, treating people fairly and respecting their autonomous choices. Moreover, many documents about what is expected of a professional will mention who a professional should be thinking of in terms of these duties, for example, patients, colleagues, and the local community. Such documents may describe the intrinsic and cooperative characteristics of a professional (see Box 9.1).

This chapter presents an approach to thinking about medical ethics and Law for healthcare professionals. The aim of the chapter is to demonstrate the presence of ethics in professionalism, and to give readers tools for identifying and reconciling ethical issues through some examples and cases.

Why bother with ethics if you can just do what the Law and professional guidelines say?

There are many reasons why a working knowledge of legal rules and professional guidelines is not necessarily enough for professional healthcare practice. Laws and guidelines can offer quite a lot of flexibility for interpretation; for example, how serious does a crime have to be before a clinician is obliged to breach a duty of confidentiality and report it? Laws and guidelines change, and change practice – we have seen this in the UK with laws that concern issues as wide ranging as abortion, bribery and candour. In some of these cases a change in the Law may create expectations and duties to which a clinician may conscientiously object.

Ethics becomes visible in a number of ways to healthcare professionals: educators may label certain contexts as ethically complex (e.g., euthanasia), there may be explicit conflict over the right thing to do, or there may just be a vague sense that something is not right. Professions may resort to a number of tools for 'doing ethics' in these situations (see Box 9.2).

Clinicians who do not understand the ethical reasons for doing things a certain way may struggle to follow a rule when it is difficult

---

ABC of Clinical Professionalism, First Edition. Edited by Nicola Cooper, Anna Frain and John Frain.
© 2018 John Wiley & Sons Ltd. Published 2018 by John Wiley & Sons Ltd.

Box 9.2 **Tools for ethical analysis.**

- **Distinguishing facts from values**; For example, 'The blood pressure is 200/100 mmHg' is a fact. That blood pressure is probably associated with an increased risk of stroke is a fact. That this is a bad blood pressure and warrants treatment funded by the state is a value judgement – look out for good, bad, right, wrong and other 'values' words.
- **Clarifying reasons and making logical arguments**: For example, 'The state has an obligation to provide free healthcare to its citizens. There are barely sufficient resources in the state-funded healthcare system for its citizens. Therefore, the state should not provide free healthcare to non-citizens'. What are the counter-arguments? Beware of false arguments (fallacies) such as 'The person making this argument is a fascist', and 'This would be the start of a slippery slope'.
- **Analysing concepts**: For example, 'If we believe that person-centred healthcare is good, then what do we understand by the terms 'person' and 'health'?'.
- **Reasoning from theory and principles**: For example, 'How can we use autonomy, beneficence, non-maleficence and justice to work out the issues in a case and then decide on the right way forward?'.
- **Comparing similar cases**: For example, 'This patient is dependent on a ventilator but is refusing this and all other medical care. How is this consistent with other cases where ventilation was or was not withdrawn, and how were those cases justified?'.
- **Thought experiments**: For example, 'If a baker had one loaf of bread and three hungry customers, how should he allocate the bread?'.

3 **Utilitarianism/Consequentialism.** This is idea of maximising good and minimising harm. The problem is how to quantify these, and what to consider a 'good' or a 'harm'. Quality adjusted life years (QALYs) are one way that the health benefits of treatments are quantified in the UK. The idea of maximising good is present in public health initiatives such as cancer screening, the collection of healthcare data and incentives for treating chronic diseases in primary care.

4 **Contractarianism.** This is the idea that without laws life would be solitary, poor, nasty, brutish and short. So society developed rights and duties, and a system of laws to protect these. Contractarian ideas apply to patients (whose rights depend on what society has agreed in terms of equitable care) and healthcare professionals (who have employment and citizenship rights in addition to duties).

Box 9.4 **Case history.**

A mother of a young child went to see her General Practitioner because of feeling depressed. During the course of the consultation it emerged that she was the victim of domestic violence, perpetrated by her partner who lived with her. She had previously attended the Emergency Department and had sustained broken bones, but had repeatedly refused to press charges. During the consultation, she asked the doctor not to breach her confidentiality and said she did not want anything to be done about her situation.

to implement (e.g., a duty of candour even when one's job may be at risk), or struggle to know what to do when there is no rule. Arguably, laws and guidelines are a form of 'procedural ethics' which have been influenced by a number of competing philosophies (see Box 9.3). Being aware of these allows for a better chance of reconciling them when they conflict.

Box 9.3 **Philosophical undercurrents in western healthcare.**

1 **Virtue Ethics.** Often attributed to the ancient Greek philosopher Aristotle, virtue ethics are popular with healthcare educators because virtue ethicists ask the question, 'How should I live?' rather than what 'What should I do?'. This idea gives rise to the characteristics of a healthcare professional such as honesty, trustworthiness, compassion and diligence. Aristotle argued that virtues were a balance of extremes – courage was at a perfect point between recklessness and cowardice. Following a number of healthcare scandals in the UK, there has been an expansion on what compassion means in healthcare and whether it is possible in pressured healthcare settings.

2 **Deontology.** Duty-based ethics based on two key ideas, that ethical duties should apply at all times, and that we should treat people always as ends in themselves and never purely as a means to an end. This means doing something because it is the right thing to do, rather than because we want to for some reason, for example, making money. Arguably, many medical codes of ethics are deontological.

The case history in Box 9.4 illustrates a difficult dilemma in which there appears to be no clear rule about what to do. Take a moment to read it.

The General Practitioner (GP) is under a professional duty where children are concerned – if a child is at risk of harm, then this overrides the interests of others. However, the GP has to consider *whether* a child is a risk, what the best approach to the situation is, and who to involve, because there is potential to trigger harm just by interfering. If there are no children involved, then it is very difficult for the GP to interfere unless he/she thinks the woman in the scenario has less autonomy in some way (e.g., her silence is because of the threat of further violence) or she is in immediate danger. Here, a duty to respect patient autonomy and confidentiality clashes with a duty to safeguard adults and children from harm. Furthermore, a duty to safeguard adults and children also includes a duty to think about the safest way to do this for the people at risk. There may be minimum duties to find out how risky the situation is and to seek advice from a relevant service (provided by the Police, social services or a domestic violence charity). There may be a minimum duty to find out if anyone is already involved in safeguarding those at risk (e.g., if the situation has been addressed in the Emergency Department). However, assuming (or hoping) that a difficult issue will be dealt with by someone else, and therefore doing nothing, is not a good approach to this case.

The case history in Box 9.5 illustrates how an ethical approach to practice can help even if doctors are not fully aware of the relevant laws and guidelines.

Box 9.5 **Case history.**

Two General Practitioner (GP) trainees were doing a mock examination for part of their membership examination. The scenario they were presented with was a completely new one for both of them: a patient attended stating he had lost his prescription for methadone (in his case, a substitute for injecting heroin). He asked for another prescription.

The first trainee saw this as an opportunity to demonstrate her skills in writing a prescription for controlled drugs. She did it quickly and clearly, writing out the dose in words and figures, and marking the prescription so it could not be altered. The second trainee considered the benefits and harms of giving a prescription in these circumstances. She was unsure whether the patient's story was genuine. She arranged for the next few doses to be taken under supervision, mindful that sudden withdrawal from opiates can be harmful and not wanting the patient to resort to using street drugs.

The trainees discussed the case afterwards and decided to find out what good practice should be in this scenario.

Recognising the Law applied to healthcare

Laws often enshrine ethical principles, and debates around whether to change or how to interpret the Law in practice are often ethical in nature. In the UK there is a hierarchy of Law (see Figure 9.1) – Law that is enacted by the Government (known as Statute Law), and Law that has developed over time as cases are used to develop the interpretation of statutes and previous cases (known as Case Law and often referred to as Common Law). Professional bodies will usually develop guidelines for practice based on Statute or Case Law.

The Law affects professionals in two key ways: (1) By defining their professional duties and boundaries (or anyone could claim to be a healthcare professional such as doctor); and (2) by establishing society's consensus on what people (including professionals) may or may not do. Box 9.6 lists a selection of key statutes with relevance to healthcare (some are general laws applied to healthcare and others are specific to the healthcare setting).

Case Law, consent and capacity

In the UK, the ways in which Law is interpreted depends on how it has been interpreted in previous cases; this is also the case in Australia and the USA. This is important when a legal principle has

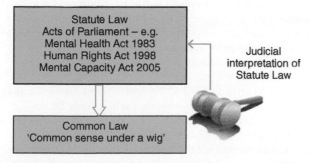

Figure 9.1 Hierarchy of Law in the UK. (N.B. Examples shown here do not necessarily apply in Scotland.)

Box 9.6 **Some UK Statute Laws with particular relevance to healthcare.**

(N.B. Examples shown here do not necessarily apply in Scotland.)

- **The Offenses Against the Person Act (1861)**: This law defines criminal offences such as assault, murder and abortion. The nature of clinical practice is that good ethical and legal practice avoids the offenses spelled out in this Act. For example, valid consent usually means that the clinician had not committed an assault.
- **The Family Law Reform Act (1969)**: This defines the age at which a person may presumed to be able to consent to medical treatment and sexual intercourse. It does not make provision for refusal of medical treatment if parents give consent.
- **The Data Protection Act (1998)**: This Act specifies how any stored personal data should be treated. A core principle is that data should only be used for the purposes for which there is explicit consent. It should also be protected from unauthorised access.
- **The Human Rights Act (1998)**: This brings the articles of the European Convention on Human Rights into British Law. It includes the right to life, the right to freedom from inhuman and degrading treatment, the right to marry and found a family, and the right to freedom of conscience and religion. These rights apply to clinicians as well as patients.
- **The Terrorism Act (2004)**: This is an example of legislation that compels clinicians to break confidentiality. Any citizen who encounters information about terrorism anywhere in the world and does not disclose it may be criminally prosecuted.
- **The Mental Capacity Act (2005)**: This legislation defines the legal principles of capacity to consent, it gives legal force to valid written advance decisions, and is for the most part the basis on which someone could be lawfully treated when capacity is absent, for example due to severe illness.
- **The Mental Health Act (amended 2007)**: The various Mental Health Acts relate to mental illness only (and not mental capacity). They produce a legal definition of mental illness and define when someone may be detained, assessed and treated for a mental health problem. Both Mental Capacity and Mental Health Acts make provision for independent advocates (if a suitable relative or friend is unavailable), to ensure that people's right to autonomy is not unnecessarily overridden.

not been clarified in a Statute. For example, prior to the Mental Capacity Act 2005, the definition of capacity relied on a case where a Court upheld the right of a man with schizophrenia to refuse the amputation of a gangrenous leg. Doctors thought an amputation would be in his best interests. The case defined the idea that if a person can understand, retain and weigh information to make a decision, then they have the right to refuse medical treatment for any or no reason.

Consent has not yet been 'tidied' by an Act of Parliament, and professional guidelines on consent rely on a series of court cases. In the most recent of these, the UK Supreme Court has stated that the person obtaining consent for medical treatment should make a reasonable attempt to find out what risks matter to that particular patient, and not withhold 'relevant information'. What is relevant is what the patient wants to know. This is different from previous legal decisions that suggested clinicians should disclose what risks would be relevant to a 'prudent' patient. Consider how this links back to the ethics: the duty to respect patient autonomy is connected to the idea that people should treat other people as 'ends in themselves' (that is, with inherent value).

Ethics and professional boundaries

Box 9.7 describes a case scenario relating to professional boundaries.

In this scenario, despite being unaware of the Data Protection Act, the trainee recognised that there was an ethical issue that needed to be addressed. Romantic liaisons between healthcare professionals and patients are considered to be unprofessional. Healthcare professionals using their status in order to gain a sexual or romantic advantage over a patient is explicitly forbidden in professional guidelines (e.g., General Medical Council: *Good Medical Practice*, 2013). This is seen as an abuse of the trust and power that is vested in the clinician while a therapeutic relationship is ongoing. In this particular scenario, the healthcare records are being used inappropriately. Boundary violations like this, however, are not the only aspect of professional boundaries worth considering. Healthcare professionals are often called upon to act in ways that blur professional boundaries, for example, acting as legal witnesses, interceding with families on behalf of patients, and treating friends or colleagues. Working within the boundaries of one's specialist skills and competence may also be challenged, for example, when doctors are asked to treat dental problems in primary care, or when someone with little training is called to help with the emergency delivery of a baby.

Conscientious objection is one area where personal beliefs and values may come into conflict with professional or occupational duties. The Law and society tolerates some instances of conscientious objection; for example, there is no obligation to be directly involved an abortion provided that the patient can seek advice elsewhere and this does not threaten the patient's immediate health or life. However, this does not mean that a clinician is expected to provide care they do not believe to be in a patient's best interests. The areas in which conscientious objection is legitimate (e.g., participation in judicial execution) is an area for debate.

Inter-professional ethics

Box 9.8 describes a case scenario relating to inter-professional ethics. The doctor and the nurse in this scenario are both acting on duty. The nurse is safeguarding all of her patients, based on the idea that interrupting the administration of medicines can result in harmful medication errors, and the doctor is responding to the clinical need of a patient in pain. Both may have been 'told' that these duties come before anything else. Clearly, there could be better mutual understanding and communication in this scenario.

Inter-professional care is when different professional groups work together to deliver healthcare that promotes the well-being of the patient. However, inter-professional working may sometimes be subject to misunderstanding, with issues such as:

- Poor communication.
- A limited understanding of others' roles and responsibilities.
- Disagreement over fair allocation of resources across/between teams.
- Different or differently nuanced values held by different staff groups who interact in the healthcare setting.

Interactions between different types of healthcare workers may generate problems that arguably have a moral dimension. Accordingly, 'inter-professional ethics' means having an approach to understanding the professional principles, social structures, and workplace processes that influence ethical aspects of inter-professional care. So, it is worth thinking about whether different professionals either have different sets of ethical principles or value them differently. Consider whether a public health doctor and a genitourinary medicine consultant might have slightly different views on the principle of confidentiality. Structures refer to the ways that different professions define their work and professional boundaries. A simplified example might be that in the UK midwives are largely concerned with normal pregnancy and obstetricians with abnormal pregnancy, which can cause conflicts when medical and midwifery students 'compete' for experience in delivering babies. Processes refers to the real world practice of medicine, in which different professionals may be labouring on behalf of the same patient but under different resources and commitments and in different settings.

Box 9.7 **Case history.**

A trainee optometrist complained to her supervisor that she struggled to have the opportunities to meet the right kind of romantic partner. She wanted to meet a fellow professional. Her supervisor listened to her description of the kind of person she would like to meet and told her that he performed an eye test for just the right person only the previous day. The client was a financial adviser. The supervisor looked up the client's details and showed them to the trainee. "Why don't you give this person a call on the pretext of some financial advice and see what happens?", he said. The trainee was uncomfortable – not only did the use of a healthcare record in this way break the Law (see Box 9.4), but it also felt unprofessional.

Box 9.8 **Case history.**

A newly qualified doctor noticed that one of the patients in a hospital ward was in pain. She established that the patient had not been given sufficient pain medication postoperatively. The doctor saw that a nurse on the ward was dispensing medications from a trolley. The nurse was wearing a tabard that stated in big letters, 'Drug round – do not interrupt'. The doctor prescribed appropriate painkillers for immediate use on the patient's drug chart and asked the nurse to dispense these. However, the nurse said, 'Do not interrupt me until I have finished'. The doctor related the story to her father, an eminent academic, who told the story in a public lecture as an example of how 'even nurses don't have compassion any more'.

Probity and professionalism – what does this mean?

Box 9.9 describes a case scenario relating to probity (a word which is synonymous with integrity). In this scenario the student who spoke up is displaying integrity. The student is consciously acting in accordance with his or her ethical duties and sense of what is right, despite pressure from a senior clinician to do something different. In this case, it helps that the student is able to say why it would be wrong to perform a rectal examination.

Box 9.9 **Case history.**

A group of medical students was taken to see a patient by surgeon. The patient had advanced dementia and was unable to say anything except, 'No'. The patient had a rectal tumour. The surgeon invited all the students in turn to perform a digital rectal examination on the patient, saying, "This is a great learning opportunity and the patient probably will not be able to remember it".

The students had a sense of unease about this situation. They had all been attentive in their medical ethics lectures about consent and capacity, but the surgeon was one of the people who marked their examination papers. One of the group, however, was able to say, "I don't think this is right. The patient is unable to consent to an intimate examination, and it is not necessary or in the patient's best interests".

To act with probity means to be trustworthy, honest, and to act with integrity. Trainees' portfolios will often have an explicit section devoted to probity. Probity is often interpreted as honesty about conflicts of interests or finances (e.g., taxes, expense claims and receiving gifts). More broadly, however, probity is about honesty and integrity in clinical practice. It is arguably easier to for clinicians to display integrity if they know what their duties are and why. Sometimes, as in the case scenario, integrity is not necessarily easy to put into practice.

Further reading/resources

British Medical Association Board of Science (2014) Ethical considerations for healthcare professionals dealing with domestic abuse, in *Domestic Abuse. BMA Board of Science Report*. BMA, London.

Hilton, S. and Slotnick, H. (2005) Proto-professionalism: how professionalisation occurs across the continuum of medical education. *Medical Education*, **39** (1), 58–65.

Toon, P. (2007) Setting Boundaries, in *Primary Care Ethics* (eds D. Bowman and J. Spicer), Radcliffe, Oxford.

Clark, P., Cott, C., and Drinka, T. (2007) Theory and practice in interprofessional ethics: a framework for understanding ethical issues in healthcare teams. *Journal of Interprofessional Care*, **21** (6), 591–603.

Papanikitas, A. (2009) Doctors should do as they are told: myth or reality? *Journal of the Royal Society of Medicine*, **102** (1), 40–42.

British Medical Association Ethics Department (2013) *Everyday Medical Ethics and Law*. BMJ Books/Wiley-Blackwell, Oxford.

CHAPTER 10

Teaching and Assessing Professionalism

John C. McLachlan[1] and Kathryn A. Robertson[2]

[1] School of Medicine, Pharmacy and Health, Durham University, Durham, UK
[2] Northern Deanery, Durham University, Durham, UK

OVERVIEW

- Professionalism is hard to define, but also hard to understand – can it be taught, can it be learned, does it develop gradually, or is it an innate personal quality?
- The professionalism 'curriculum' can be formal (intended), informal (opportunistic) and hidden (arising from the cultural context).
- Assessment of professionalism may be subjective (assessed by observers) or objective (assessed by performance on written materials).
- Hazards arise in both approaches.

"Can you tell me, Socrates, whether virtue is acquired by teaching or by practice; or if neither by teaching nor practice, then whether it comes to man by nature, or in what other way?"

Plato, Dialogues.

Introduction

Medical professionalism is important but hard to define. It is interpreted differently in different historical periods, in different cultural and geographic settings, in different individuals, and in the same individuals in different contexts. However, it is as important as knowledge and skills in ensuring good patient care.

We identify four different lenses through which doctors view the practice of medicine (Figure 10.1). The 'profession' lens suffers from the challenges listed in the preceding paragraph. The 'vocation' lens may lead doctors to drive themselves too hard, to be too self-abnegating in the face of the demands of medicine. The 'job' lens might, for instance, lead a doctor to feel that they should be able to finish work at the end of their shift, and that responsibility for providing adequate ongoing care lies with their employer, and the 'career' lens may lead junior doctors who witness unprofessionalism in seniors to feel coerced into tacitly complying, for fear of repercussions.

In its positive aspects, medical professionalism is associated with good patient care. It is predictable from early career stages. Faculty assessments predict future professionalism performance as assessed by later 'Fitness to Practice' censures (high scores mean a low likelihood of successful disciplinary action), but oddly, so do examination results (where high scores also predict a low likelihood of successful disciplinary action). This is surprising, since we do not normally think of 'exam performance' and 'positive moral and ethical qualities' as being related.

It is important to appreciate that the environment – in terms of resources, workloads and organisational culture – plays a key role in mediating professional behaviour.

It is important to state that *attitudes* are not observable: only external *behaviours* are. A key unresolved issue is the question of whether constrained behaviour is eventually internalized – does a sexist surgeon who is required by the environment to behave in non-sexist ways eventually become less sexist? And how does *what you know you should do*, and *what you do whilst being assessed*, relate to *what you actually do* when you are not observed? Finally, other internal states may affect behaviour; how a doctor behaves after a week of night shifts may be different from how she or he behaves after a week's holiday.

Becoming professional

There is uncertainty about how professionalism develops (see Figure 10.2). The conventional view is that it can be taught: that as trainees embark on their training programme they are not yet professionals, and that they will move through a stage of being proto-professional to true professionalism because of the teaching they are given. In this conscious learning model, trainees study professionalism and act on the results of their studies. However, there are other possibilities. One is that professionalism is 'caught' like a disease, through the close proximity of more senior practitioners, and is therefore learned tacitly. A further possibility is that professionalism derives from a stable personality characteristic, either innate or set during childhood. This could either be evident at the

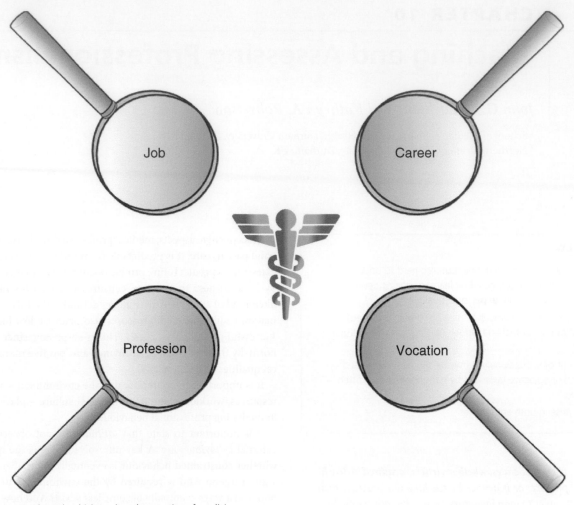

Figure 10.1 Lenses through which to view the practice of medicine.

beginning of the training period, or be developmental, revealing itself as the trainee matures.

The distinctions between these possibilities are significant. If professionalism is learnt, we have a problem of teaching: if it is innate, we have a problem of selection.

In a number of studies, student professionalism seems to decline over the course of the undergraduate programme. This is worrying, because it suggests either that the teaching is making things worse, or that it is failing to counteract other factors that are making it worse.

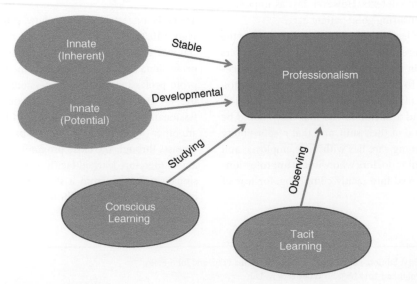

Figure 10.2 Ways in which professionalism may develop.

A related issue is that of professional identity formation. Professions construct identities that may differ radically from 'official' descriptions of themselves.

The curriculum

There are also different versions of the 'curriculum' (Figure 10.3). The formal curriculum is that which is intended to be delivered by the organisation – for instance, by the medical school. However, what is *actually* delivered may not match the intention, and the student experience may be differ significantly (if students do not attend all sessions, for instance). Assessment is a key part of the formal curriculum.

The informal curriculum represents opportunistic encounters between teachers and learners, where the nature of the learning is spontaneous and context-specific, and hence unplanned, even if the encounters are programmed. Nonetheless, there is still intentionality in creating such opportunities.

Finally, there is the hidden curriculum, not intended by either the formal or informal curricula. This is the consequence of working within and observing the community of practice, and represents the unwritten (perhaps even unspoken) social and cultural values of the community. The hidden curriculum is assimilated through observing 'what actually happens', and enforced through social norms. There may be positive lessons to learn from such observations but, because of the process of professional identity formation, the culture of the environment or the resource constraints, there may also be negative aspects to the hidden curriculum. It can have a very considerable impact on the learner because it appears authentic, and negative role modelling can have profound unfortunate consequences. A number of studies indicate that negative modelling of professionalism (for instance, bullying) is dependent on local culture, particularly local leadership.

The formal curriculum may be delivered through 'classroom' teaching. Aspects of professionalism which may be delivered in this way include knowledge of relevant law, ethics, guidelines and policies in the organisations in which healthcare is being delivered. There may be professional codes of practice such as the General Medical Council's *Good Medical Practice* and *Duties of a Doctor* to explicate. Patient confidentiality, consent and end-of-life care, for instance, are perhaps best introduced as concepts in formal teaching.

The informal curriculum may include experiential teaching and learning in simulated or real settings. Generally, in informal settings, at least one team member is a health professional, and the settings are authentic. There may be structured opportunities to offer and receive feedback.

Barriers to learning

There are challenges to the teaching and learning of professionalism. One barrier is that students (and sometimes teachers) may rate professionalism as less important than knowledge or skills. Professionalism may therefore not be adequately represented in the curriculum.

As students approach clinical practice, pressure to demonstrate knowledge and skills that align with those of the community may increase, and professionalism may not be seen as an undoubted key attribute. Perhaps this contributes to the declines in measured professionalism during training seen in many environments. Examples of unprofessional behaviour on the part of seniors as part of the hidden curriculum may also play a role.

Assessments

It is too simplistic to say that 'assessment drives learning', as it could also be said that 'assessment drives cheating' and 'assessment inhibits learning' in some circumstances. A strong case can also be made that role modelling and the hidden curriculum drive learning, even when this runs contrary to the taught and assessed curricula. However, assessment is certainly a contributor to student behaviour, and a marker for the importance the organisation attaches to professionalism.

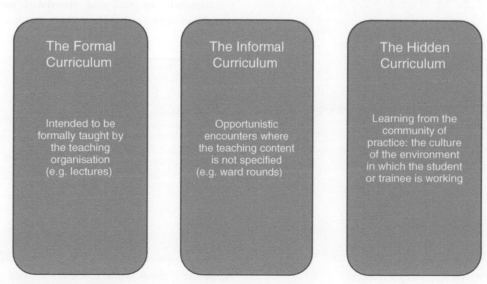

Figure 10.3 Different varieties of 'the curriculum'.

Good assessments are valid, reliable, practical, acceptable and defensible

Good assessments are valid, reliable, practical, acceptable and defensible (see Figure 10.4). A *valid* assessment is one that measures what you want it to measure. *Reliability* has a special technical meaning: it specifically means *does the assessment measure consistently? Acceptability* is important too, in that both candidates and assessors have to agree that an assessment is worthwhile in order for them to work on their respective tasks, rather than candidates looking for short cuts which do not involve actual learning, and assessors just 'ticking boxes'. *Practicality* has cost (particularly in assessor time) as a key consideration, but scalability and generalisability are also factors. A method of exploring professionalism may work well in a pilot study, but may be impossible to apply to a larger setting. *Defensibility* means that the assessment will stand up to challenge, both within the organisation, and legally.

Assessments: formative or summative?

Assessments can be either formative (intended to help the candidate improve) or summative (intended to aid in progression decisions about the candidate). While summative outcomes may have formative consequences (failing an assessment should tell the candidate something important), formative assessments should never have summative consequences, and indeed, assessments should be designed separately for each of these purposes. Both types of assessment should have a positive educational impact in terms of how candidates approach learning. For instance, in Objective Structured Clinical Examinations (OSCEs) we generally require candidates to carry out tasks within a very strict and short time frame. If candidates learn to carry out the procedures quickly but not thoroughly, the OSCE could have a negative educational impact. Objective measures are usually summative, while subjective measures may be either formative or summative.

Assessments: subjective or objective?

Assessment methods may be categorised into subjective and objective approaches (see Figure 10.5). Subjective methods rely on a decision by an individual, where another individual might well come to a different decision. These are most clearly recognised in observational methods such as MiniCEX (clinical examination scenarios) and DOPS (direct observation of practical skills) (see below). Even OSCEs are not truly objective in nature, despite the name. Indeed, it is possible in healthcare settings for the variability introduced by assessors to be greater than the variability of the candidates. Subjective measures essentially rely on observation and report. These measures may have individual low reliability, but are assumed to have high validity. A key aspect of subjective approaches is who makes the subjective decision.

Objective methods remove the observer from the scoring process. Examples are given below, but generally involve computer scoring of some kind. This significantly improves reliability, but may raise questions about validity. Objective tests are frequently associated with the formal component of the curriculum.

Subjective assessments

Subjective assessments can be categorised by those who carry them out:

- **'Tutor'-led assessment**: Here, we use 'tutor' to include all those with formal responsibility for teaching and assessment; hence, faculty, staff and educational and clinical supervisors. Tutor-led assessments include OSCEs, and work-based assessments such as MiniCEX and DOPs.
- **Peer assessment**: A disadvantage of 'tutor'-based observational methods is that the candidates know they are under observation. Their behaviours may not correspond to what they actually do in practice when not observed. In addition, tutors are able to observe learners on only a limited number of occasions. In many ways, peers are the best observers of professionalism, since they see each other's uncensored behaviour in a wide range of settings. Unfortunately, when summative judgements are to be made, peer group loyalty generally exceeds adherence to professionalism and peers may collude to subvert the process, and/or 'fail to fail'.
- **Assessment by real and simulated patients**: A valuable addition to professionalism assessment is scoring by simulated

Good assessments are:

- Valid (measures what you want to measure)
- Reliable (measures consistently)
- Acceptable (trainees and assessors are prepared to co-operate in the process)
- Practical (can be delivered at reasonable cost at time scales)
- Defensible (will stand up to challenges, including legal challenges)

Figure 10.4 The attributes of a high-quality assessment.

Objective	Subjective
Knowledge, exams	Tutor ratings (including OSCEs etc.)
Number of resits	Peer ratings
Situational judgement tests	Self ratings
Personal qualities	Patient ratings
Assessments	Multisource feedback
Conscientiousness Index	Exception reporting
	Portfolios
	MiniPEX

Figure 10.5 A classification of assessment methods.

patients and genuine patients who have received some training in how to approach the task. Simulated patients who have been trained in their role offer the possibility of consistency in presentation between students, while real patients offer authenticity of experience.

- **Self-assessment**: Some approaches require candidates to assess themselves as part of the professionalism process, perhaps as part of a portfolio process (see below). Sadly, the evidence suggests that self-assessment is not reliable: a particular problem is candidates who are 'incompetent and unaware'.
- **Multisource feedback**: All of the above can be combined in '360-degree evaluation' or 'multisource feedback (MSF), where a wide variety of colleagues at all levels express an anonymous view. Literature suggests that MSF can bring about performance improvement, but it is valuable to give structured feedback on the outcomes, rather than just the raw results. This increases costs significantly.
- **Exception reporting (critical incidents)**: While professionalism is difficult to define, many feel that they can recognise its absence. This is the basis for exception reporting, where a particular (generally negative) incident is observed and recorded in a specific context. This is particularly valuable when a pattern of incidents emerges, each of which alone may be insufficient to trigger 'fitness to practice' action but together suggest cause for concern. However, by its nature, exception reporting is a relatively unusual event; hence, this approach cannot be used to assess all members of a cohort for professionalism.
- **Portfolios**: These represent aggregations of events described by the candidates, and may include logs of training, learning experiences and patient encounters, reports of assessment outcomes, feedback from colleagues and patients, self-reported critical incidents, and reflective writing, among other components. They are widely viewed as a way of gaining insight into professional attributes. Interestingly, despite their widespread introduction and use in summative settings such as the UK's Annual Review of Competence Progression (ARCP), evidence on their predictive validity is sparse.

Objective assessments

Objective assessments consist of the following:

- **Examination items**: It is straightforward to test for declarative knowledge of relevant laws, guidelines and ethical principles relating to professional practice, through MCQs. Evidently, if candidates do not know the rules and guidelines, then they cannot follow them (even though knowing what they are does not mean that candidates *will* follow them). Such tests are highly reliable. As noted earlier, knowledge examinations and number of re-sits also predict later professional clinical practice.
- **Situational judgement tests (SJTs)**: These are scenario-based items that require candidates to select the course of action that they *should* take (as opposed to *would* take). In selection, it has been demonstrated that they have better predictive validity than interviews. A key question is what SJTs are testing, since they are not directly testing knowledge or skills. One possibility is that they are testing Implicit Trait Policies, which represent aspects of behaviour learned earlier in life. It is therefore plausible that they

are testing aspects that relate strongly to subsequent 'professional' behaviours.

- **The Conscientiousness Index**: We noted previously that both subjective professionalism ratings and objective knowledge examination scores positively predict later professional practice as assessed via disciplinary proceedings.

Conscientiousness Index

We have theorised that examination results predict professionalism in future medical practice due to the presence of a common personality factor. Within the 'Five Factor' personality model (Openness to new experience, Conscientiousness, Agreeableness, Extraversion, and Neuroticism), conscientiousness is known from non-medical work psychology studies to be the strongest single predictor of workplace performance, and is an important factor in medical student success.

We have proposed that the common factor between high examination scores and low probability of subsequent censure is the trait of *conscientiousness* – candidates who are conscientious are likely to receive high professional ratings, but are also likely to attend teaching and training sessions and therefore do well in assessments of knowledge and skills. Conscientiousness in minor matters in training environments may well be predictive of conscientiousness in later clinical settings such as keeping good patient notes, keeping up to date, following up on patient referrals, and so forth.

We developed a Conscientiousness Index (CI), initially for medical students, and have been able to show that in a variety of settings it co-distributes with independent staff and peer ratings of professionalism. The CI is constructed from serial objective measures of properties such as bringing complete induction information, attending compulsory sessions and completing administrative requirements. Not only is the CI objective and scalar but it is also low cost, since virtually all the data are already recorded in one setting or another. All that is required is to bring it together in one place. The CI has been successfully extended to postgraduate medicine and to other healthcare professions, although the exact nature of the components of the CI obviously depends on the particular context. A list of example components which have emerged from various workshops on the CI at international conferences is shown in Figure 10.6. Normally, a CI would use four or five of these components, but it could be less or more. New components could be added to suit particular circumstances, as long as they are objective 'yes–no' items, rather than subjective judgement calls.

Box 10.1 shows a typical distribution of CI scores, and describes what the likely consequences might be.

Failure to fail

A significant issue in the assessment of professionalism is the phenomenon of 'failure to fail', where observers 'pass' candidates who they really believe should fail. Reasons for this include concern about the future of the individual, compliance with colleagues' estimations or institutional policy, doubts about the assessment process or their own adequacy as a teacher or assessor and, perhaps most importantly, concerns about what will happen to themselves if they fail a student – will there be anger, tears, appeals, challenges, or even accusations of bias and prejudice?

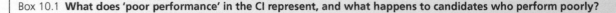

Attendance information

Attending compulsory sessions
Attending punctually (defining punctual)
Signing in and out of sessions
Notification of absence
Attending agreed meetings
Proper notice for rota change requests

Induction information

Submitting employment requirements
(visas etc.)
Bringing required ID
Bringing photographs
Criminal convictions information
Immunisation record up to date

Assessment data

Submitting assignments on time
Completing and collecting information
(e.g. portfolios)
Complying with assessment requirements

Teaching and learning data

Collecting required course materials
Collecting marked log books
Accessing the Virtual Learning
Environment
Completing compulsory on line modules

Administrative data

Logging duty hours appropriately
Attending administrative organisation
sessions

Evaluation information

Completing unit evaluations
Responding to on line polls

Figure 10.6 Possible components of a Conscientiousness Index.

Box 10.1 **What does 'poor performance' in the CI represent, and what happens to candidates who perform poorly?**

Invariably in our studies, the distribution of CI scores is a skewed normal distribution with a long tail, as shown below.

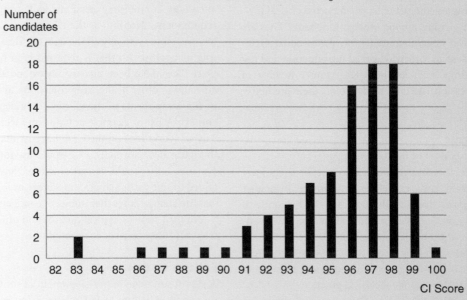

Concerns arise with those in the long tail, rather than those in the main distribution. There are two possibilities for addressing these students.

Formative responses

While we believe that conscientiousness is a relatively stable trait, there is some evidence that formative feedback on lack of conscientious performance in everyday tasks can have positive effects. Junior doctors have been shown to improve their compliance with administrative tasks when their scores are shown to them.

Summative responses

We are now sufficiently confident in the CI to also use it for summative purposes. First, the distribution of CI scores is reviewed to confirm that it shows the standard 'long tail of responses', where some candidates are performing markedly less well than the norm. These candidates (2 standard deviations below the year mean) are reviewed individually for factors, such as illness or disability, that might legitimately have affected their engagement with the course. In the absence of such factors, these candidates lose one professionalism 'life' out of a possible five. The other four are their tutor professionalism rating, their portfolio score, their family project and reflective writing score, and the presence of two or more critical incident forms. Loss of two or more 'lives' means that the Professionalism Domain has been failed. Students may successfully remediate this over the summer by reflective writing on why they failed, have to repeat the year, or have their studies terminated.

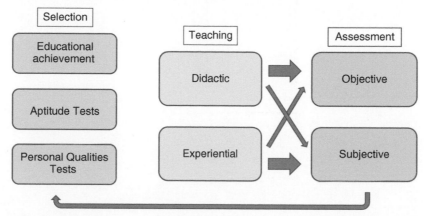

Figure 10.7 Didactic taught material may be best assessed by objective means such as written examinations and experiential development by subjective observations, but there is some cross over between the two. Assessment links back to selection to indicate that the most important thing may be to choose the right candidates initially.

Selection

Earlier we posed the question as to whether professionalism was innate rather than acquired, and therefore represented partly an issue of selection rather than education. The traditional interview and responses to personal statements have been shown to be poor predictors of later performance. The strongest predictor in most settings is prior educational performance. However, Multiple Mini Interviews, SJTs and tests of cognitive abilities have been shown to have valuable predictive validity for later clinical performance (see Figure 10.7).

Further reading/resources

Thistlethwaite, J. and Spencer, J. (2008) *Professionalism in Medicine*. CRC Press, Boca Raton.

Stern, D.T. (2006) *Measuring Medical Professionalism*. Oxford University Press, Oxford.

Thistlethwaite, J. and McKimm, J. (2015) *Health Care Professionalism at a Glance*. Wiley Blackwell.

Cruess, R.L. and Cruess, S.R. (2006) Teaching professionalism: general principles. *Medical Teacher*, **28**, 205–208.

Cleland, J.A., Knight, L.V., Rees, C.E., Tracey, S. and Bond C.M. (2008) Is it me or is it them? Factors that influence the passing of underperforming students. *Medical Education*, **42**, 800–809.

Margolis, E. (ed.) (2001) *The Hidden Curriculum in Higher Education*. Routledge, New York.

Kelly, M., O'Flynn, S., McLachlan, J. and Sawdon, M.A. (2012) The clinical conscientiousness index: A valid tool for exploring professionalism in the clinical undergraduate setting. *Academic Medicine*, **87**, 1218–1224.

McLachlan, J.C. (2006) The relationship between assessment and learning. *Medical Education*, **40**, 716–717.

Patterson, F., Zibarras, L. and Ashworth, V. (2016) Situational judgement tests in medical education and training: Research, theory and practice. *Medical Teacher*, **38**, 3–17.

CHAPTER 11

Regulation of Healthcare Professionals

John Alcolado[1] and Clare Sutherland[2]

[1] Division of Medical Sciences and Graduate Entry Medicine, University of Nottingham, UK
[2] Derby Teaching Hospitals NHS Foundation Trust, Derby, UK

OVERVIEW

- Healthcare professionals are regulated by Law – only someone with the appropriate training and qualifications who is registered to practise can work as a doctor, nurse or allied health professional.
- Regulation is underpinned by the concept of professionalism.
- Regulators set professional standards that practitioners should follow, and oversee systems that ensure they continue to meet these standards.
- Regulators investigate complaints about individual practitioners; investigations can include assessments of performance.
- Regulators can take action to prevent practitioners putting the safety of patients, or the public's confidence in the profession, at risk.

Introduction

Governments and States have a legitimate interest in exercising authority, control and oversight of key economic and socio-political activities. In general, the more vital the service, the greater will be the pressure from citizens to ensure it is properly regulated, and the greater will be the temptation for politicians to exert influence. Healthcare is one example.

The regulation of healthcare can be broadly divided into the regulation of organisations that provide services (e.g., hospitals, clinics and private companies) and the regulation of individual practitioners who work independently or within these organisations. In England, the Care Quality Commission (CQC) inspects organisations that provide healthcare. Other interested parties include Royal Colleges (which set professional standards), Health Education England (which delivers education and training), and other regulatory bodies (see Figure 11.1). Similar arrangements exist in the devolved nations of Scotland, Wales and Northern Ireland.

Individual practitioners are regulated by the General Medical Council (GMC), General Dental Council (GDC), the Nursing and Midwifery Council (NMC) and others. Some groups of healthcare workers (e.g., healthcare assistants, physicians' associates and health service managers) are not regulated. A full list of UK healthcare professions regulators is given in Box 11.1. The Professional Standards Authority for Health and Social Care is the overarching regulator that oversees the function of these regulatory bodies.

Regulation is underpinned by the concept of professionalism. This chapter outlines how regulation applies to healthcare professionals in the UK, which is similar to other developed countries. A comparison of other countries can be found in Further reading/resources.

Regulatory frameworks

A number of UK statutes give regulators the authority to oversee and control individuals practising in specific professions. The title 'doctor', when used in the context of providing healthcare, is protected and individuals may not practise medicine unless they are registered by the GMC. This is the same for nurses, social workers, and the other professions listed in Box 11.1. Complexities can arise when individuals with a doctoral qualification work in healthcare in non-medical roles – so, for example, a person with a PhD could use 'Dr' in terms of their title but they are required to take care not to imply they hold a general medical qualification if they do not.

Healthcare regulators are responsible for setting educational standards, accrediting courses in universities, and admitting individuals on to their registers. Inclusion on a professional register grants individuals a particular status and benefits. However, these are accompanied by duties and responsibilities to maintain the professional standards expected by other members of the profession and the public in general. Historically, professions were self-regulating. It is now recognised that, while specialist input is essential, public confidence in a profession can only be maintained when the public are manifestly involved in its regulation. Regulators, after due consultation, have the authority to explicitly state the standards required of healthcare practitioners (see Further reading/resources). Not everyone will agree with all the standards, but the price to be paid for belonging to a profession is adherence to the requirements set out by the regulator.

ABC of Clinical Professionalism, First Edition. Edited by Nicola Cooper, Anna Frain and John Frain.
© 2018 John Wiley & Sons Ltd. Published 2018 by John Wiley & Sons Ltd.

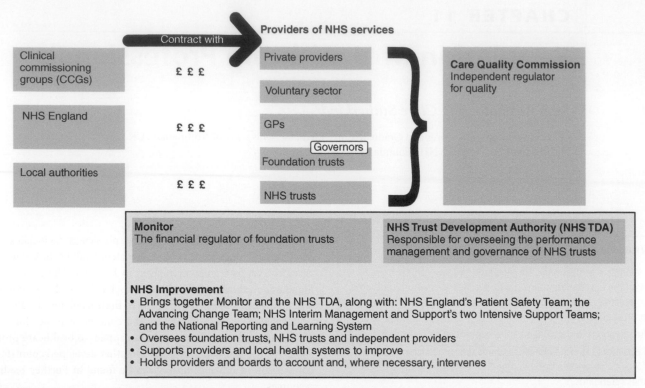

Figure 11.1 Regulatory organisations in the English NHS. Responsibility for regulating healthcare in the NHS is mainly through the *Care Quality Commission* and *NHS Improvement*. However, there are also several other authorities charged with regulating specific aspects of care, for example, the Medicines and Healthcare products Regulatory Agency (MHRA) and the Human Fertilisation and Embryology Authority (HFEA).

Box 11.1 **UK health and social care regulators.**

Regulator	Professional group
General Medical Council	Doctors
General Dental Council	Dentists, clinical dental technicians, dental hygienists, dental nurses, dental technicians, dental therapists, and orthodontic therapists
Nursing and Midwifery Council	Nurses and midwives
General Optical Council	Opticians, optometrists and dispensing opticians
General Pharmaceutical Council	Pharmacists, pharmacy technicians and pharmacy premises in England, Scotland and Wales
General Osteopathic Council	Osteopaths
General Chiropractic Council	Chiropractors
Health and Care Professions Council	Arts therapists, biomedical scientists, chiropodists/podiatrists, clinical scientists, dieticians, hearing aid dispensers, occupational therapists, operating department practitioners, orthoptists, paramedics, physiotherapists, practitioner psychologists, prosthetists/orthoptists, radiographers, social workers in England, and speech and language therapists
Care Council for Wales	Qualified social workers, and social work students on degree courses in Wales
Scottish Social Services Council	Qualified social workers, and social work students on degree courses in Scotland
Northern Ireland Social Services Council	Qualified social workers, and social work students on degree courses in Northern Ireland
Pharmaceutical Society of Northern Ireland	Pharmacists and pharmacy premises in Northern Ireland

Definition of fitness to practise

A key function of a regulator is to determine whether an individual is 'fit to practise'. A regulator may remove or restrict an individual's ability to practise within a regulated profession if there is sufficient evidence of deficient performance, misconduct, adverse physical or mental health, a criminal conviction, deficient knowledge of the English language or an adverse determination by another regulatory body in the UK or overseas. These can be summarised as serious departures from the knowledge, skills and behaviours expected of a member of the profession (see Box 11.2).

If an individual behaves in a way that might call their fitness to practise into question, the regulator has powers to investigate and, if the allegations are found proved, to order a sanction. A full discussion of the legislative framework is outside the scope of this chapter, but key laws and statutes are listed in Box 11.3.

Sources and number of complaints

There has been a considerable rise in complaints to regulators during the past decade (see Box 11.4). The reasons behind this are complex but include an increased willingness by members of the public to complain, increased media interest in high-profile NHS failures, and greater publicity of the mechanisms available to complain. Complaints may be made by patients, their relatives or carers,

---

Box 11.2 **The meaning of fitness to practise (doctors).**

Doctors have a respected position in society and their work gives them privileged access to patients, some of whom may be very vulnerable. A doctor whose conduct has shown that he or she cannot justify the trust placed in him/her should not continue in unrestricted practice while that remains the case. The public is entitled to expect that their doctor is fit to practise and follows the principles described in *Good Medical Practice*.

All human beings make mistakes from time to time. Doctors are no different. While occasional one-off mistakes need to be thoroughly investigated by those immediately involved and any harm put right, they are unlikely in themselves to indicate a fitness to practise problem. However, serious or persistent failures to follow *Good Medical Practice* will put your registration at risk.

A question of fitness to practise is likely to arise if:

- A doctor's [persistent] performance has harmed patients or put patients at risk of harm.
- A doctor has shown a deliberate or reckless disregard of clinical responsibilities towards patients.
- A doctor's health is compromising patient safety.
- A doctor has abused a patient's trust or violated a patient's autonomy or other fundamental rights.
- A doctor has behaved dishonestly, fraudulently or in a way designed to mislead or harm others.

The advice above is only illustrative of the sort of behaviour which could call registration into question. The outcome in any case will depend on its particular facts.

From the GMC's *The Meaning of Fitness to Practice*, 2014. www.gmc-uk.org.

Box 11.3 **Key UK healthcare legislation relevant to regulation.**

- The Medical Act 1983 (established the General Medical Council and its powers).
- The Dentists Act 1984.
- The Opticians Act 1989.
- The Osteopaths Act 1989.
- Nursing and Midwifery Order 2001 (established the Nursing Midwifery Council and its powers).
- National Health Service Reform and Healthcare Professions Act 2002 (created the Council for the Regulation of Health Care Professionals).
- Health and Social Care Act 2012 (reorganised some of the existing regulatory frameworks).

Box 11.4 **Number of fitness to practise enquiries to the GMC by year.**

Year	No. of complaints received	Fitness to practise hearings	No. of doctors erased from the register
2014	9624	237	71
2013	9866	229	55
2012	10347	216	55
2011	8781	212	65
2010	7153	314	73
2009	5773	319	68
2008	5195	359	42
2007	5168	196	60

---

other professionals, institutions such as hospitals, members of public, the Police, or anonymously.

There is still some confusion regarding the role of the different regulators in the mind of the public. Some complaints are made to the GMC or NMC when the concerns are regarding the actions of institutions or organisations rather than specific individuals. Others contact the regulator when local investigation and informal resolution would be quicker and more appropriate.

The increasing number of complaints has resulted in considerable delays in investigations and adjudications. Such delays can be unfair to both practitioners and complainants. Regulators have responded by increasing resources and streamlining their processes. However, ultimately the cost of investigations and adjudications are met by members of the profession through increases in registration fees, and regulators need to strike a balance between the resources required for rapid and robust resolution and the fees charged to practitioners.

Separation of powers

A significant concern that has been raised regarding the regulation system in the UK is that the same organisation is often responsible for setting standards, investigating alleged breaches of those standards, charging individuals, presenting the evidence and, to some extent, determining guilt and deciding the sanction. Some attempts have been made to resolve these potential conflicts. For example, the Medical Practitioner Tribunal Service (MPTS) was set up as an independent branch of the GMC specifically to adjudicate on charges brought by the GMC. However, the MPTS remains part of the GMC and tribunal panel members are GMC associates.

The investigation process

Once a complaint is received by a regulator, a sifting process is carried out. Some are returned to the complainant because they clearly fall outside the scope of the regulator (see Box 11.5). In other cases, the regulator may ask for a local investigation and attempted resolution. It will open an investigation of any outstanding complaints or concern.

It is important to note that an investigation by a regulator will focus on the entire practice of an individual and need not be limited to the complaint itself. The regulator is seeking evidence as to whether fitness to practice may be impaired, and this may touch on issues or concerns not raised by the initial complaint. Failure to appreciate this may cause antagonism from professionals who may feel the regulator is 'trawling' for additional concerns to build a case against them. For example, the GMC will write to all known employers of a doctor asking them to provide details of any concerns that have been raised in the past. Practitioners sometimes express concerns that the regulator will investigate adverse comments in great detail, while dismissing positive comments. However, there needs to be an understanding that fundamentally the role of regulator is to protect patients, promote public safety and defend the reputation of a profession.

Regulators must act in a fair, timely and proportionate manner throughout the investigation process. Investigations can be highly stressful and can have devastating consequences for those being investigated (see Further reading/resources). Practitioners are strongly advised to obtain formal representation and avail themselves of support services (e.g., their trade union or defence organisation). In many cases the complaint and its resulting investigation

---

Box 11.5 **Complaints that fall outside the scope of the regulator.**

In general, the role of a regulator is to:

- Decide who is qualified to work in the UK.
- Set the standards that healthcare professionals should follow.
- Make sure they continue to meet these standards.
- Take action to prevent them from putting the safety of patients, or the public's confidence in the profession, at risk.

The regulator will re-direct complaints that are outside its jurisdiction – complaints about other professions, complaints about a healthcare organisation (e.g., a hospital), complaints about disagreement with a professional's opinion, and so forth. Regulators are interested in concerns that mean a professional may not be fit to practise.

Box 11.6 **Health concerns, such as drug and alcohol misuse.**

A 40-year-old General Practitioner was admitted to hospital with a seizure due to delirium tremens (alcohol withdrawal). He required at least a week in hospital before he was orientated. His father confirmed he was a regular heavy drinker. When the diagnosis was explained to him by the treating physician, he denied that alcohol was the cause for his symptoms. He stated that his car was vital for his work. He continued to deny he had an alcohol problem while he was in hospital.

The treating physician explained that the patient could not drive by Law and that he would write to the Driving and Vehicle Licensing Authority to inform them, since the patient had indicated he would continue to drive. The treating physician also explained that since the patient was also a doctor, his alcohol dependence could impair his fitness to practise and that he should seek help. On the basis that the doctor had no insight in to his health problem and did not want to seek help, he was referred to the GMC.

---

does not lead to removal of registration, but the regulator may put measures in place to support an individual back to good practice. Hence, professionals who demonstrate insight, remorse and the ability to reflect on their practice are more likely to be able to remain in their profession compared with those who do not. Health concerns, including drug and alcohol misuse, are examples where the regulator may request a medical assessment and impose restrictions on the individual's practice in order to safeguard patients (see Box 11.6).

During the initial investigation phase, the regulator will write to the professional, disclosing their concerns and asking for a response. Once any responses are received, the regulator will make a decision as to whether a health or performance assessment is required, whether to issue a warning, or charge the individual and refer the case to a fitness to practise hearing.

Interim orders

The investigation process can be time-consuming, and there is often a further delay until a case can be scheduled for a full hearing. In theory, individuals could continue in unrestricted practise during this time. The 'interim orders' system was established to allow the GMC to impose conditions or suspend the registration of a doctor pending investigation and a full fitness to practise determination. The role of interim orders tribunals is not to find facts or resolve conflicts of evidence but to carry out a risk assessment. The test is whether an interim order is necessary on the grounds of public safety, otherwise in the public interest or in the interest of the practitioner. Any interim orders must be proportionate and be the least restrictive whilst addressing the risks identified. The NMC and General Dental Council also have interim order processes.

Fitness to practise hearing and adjudication

At the end of the investigatory process, if the regulator forms the view that there is a realistic prospect that an individual's fitness to practise is impaired, it will formulate charges and proceed with a formal hearing. The burden of proof is on the regulator, and the standard of proof is the civil one – that is, the balance of probabilities.

A fitness to practise hearing is an adversarial system, as in a Court, with the regulator laying evidence against the practitioner and the practitioner submitting the defence. Civil rules of evidence apply and the decision is made by at least three panel or tribunal members, at least one of whom is a professional member and one a lay member.

Figures 11.2 and 11.3 outline the fitness to practise procedures of the GMC and NMC, and are similar to those of other healthcare regulatory bodies.

Impairment

Healthcare professionals make mistakes and will not always meet the high expectations they place on themselves, let alone those expected by the public, the media and regulators. A single act may sometimes be serious enough to cast doubt on an individual's fitness to practise, but fitness to practise usually arises when there is a pattern of persistent unacceptable behaviour.

The decision for the regulator is whether, taking all factors into consideration, an individual's knowledge, skills or behaviours

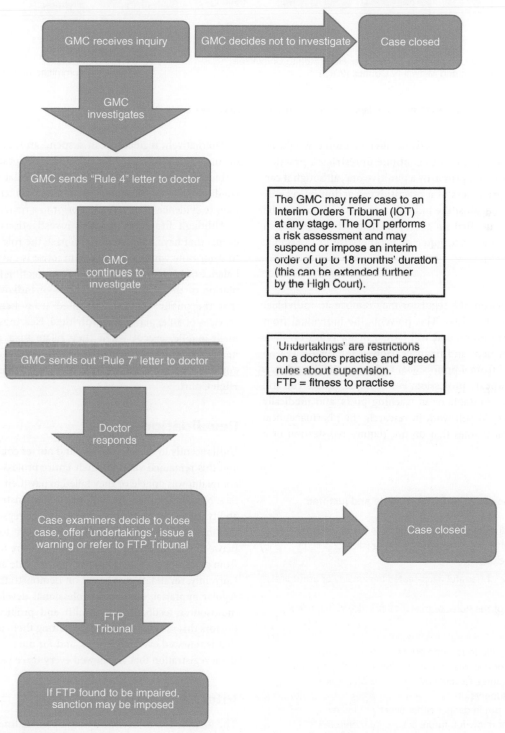

Figure 11.2 GMC fitness to practise procedures.

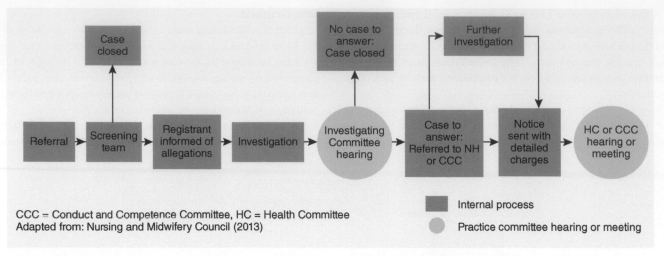

CCC = Conduct and Competence Committee, HC = Health Committee
Adapted from: Nursing and Midwifery Council (2013)

Internal process

Practice committee hearing or meeting

Figure 11.3 NMC Fitness to practise procedures. Adapted from The Nursing and Midwifery Council (2103).

are such that a properly informed member of public would be affronted if they were allowed to continue unrestricted practice. The regulator's role is not primarily a punitive one, although it can signal the inappropriateness of a practitioner's action by recording a formal finding against the individual. Any sanction must be proportionate and justified on the basis that it is necessary to protect the public, the practitioner, or is otherwise in the public interest (see Box 11.7).

Sanctions

As an ultimate sanction, the regulator may remove an individual from the professional register. This prevents the individual from working in their profession and will have a major effect on their self-esteem, employment and finances. However, individuals who have been removed from a professional register can still work in a non-regulated healthcare profession. For example, nurses can still work as healthcare assistants or in teaching posts, and medically qualified doctors could still work in research, the pharmaceutical industry or in clinical roles that do not require registration or a licence to practise.

Box 11.7 **Sanctions must be proportionate and justified.**

The NMC has published guidelines on the type of things panels should consider when they are deciding if a sanction should be imposed. These include:

- Is there evidence of harmful deep-seated personality or attitudinal problems?
- Are there areas of the nurse or midwife's practice which need retraining?
- Is there evidence of general incompetence?
- Is there a willingness to respond positively to retraining?
- Does the nurse or midwife accept they have a health problem and are prepared to agree to abide by conditions on medical treatment and supervision?
- Will patients be put in danger either directly or indirectly?
- Can the nurse or midwife's future actions be monitored?

Alternatively, regulators can suspend an individual for a period of time. This sends a strong signal that the practitioner has fallen seriously below the standards expected. Regulators can also impose conditions on registration, place limits on clinical practice, or require evidence of remediation prior to a review hearing.

Although fitness to practise investigations are triggered by events that have happened in the past, the role of the regulator is to determine whether fitness to practise is currently impaired. A balance needs to be struck between protecting the public, the reputation of the profession, the rights of individual, and ensuring that the public are not prevented from benefitting from the services of an experienced individual. Hearings and decisions are made public, except when they relate to a practitioner's own health issues. Because regulation of healthcare professionals is governed by statute, appeals against sanctions are made to the High Court.

Revalidation

Until recently in the UK, doctors and nurses could gain registration and this remained valid for their entire professional lives, unless a complaint was upheld or they failed to pay their annual registration fees. Now, individuals are required to demonstrate their continued ability to practise in order to remain on the register through 'revalidation'. The revalidation process attempts to strike a balance between the resources required and the desire to protect the public from practitioners who do not keep up to date and may pose a risk. Currently, revalidation is based on demonstrating participation in regular appraisal, continual professional development, reflection, multisource feedback, and health and probity declarations. For doctors this results in the GMC granting them a licence to practise that is renewed every five years, and for nurses the NMC granting them registration that is renewed every three years.

International factors

The jurisdiction of healthcare regulators is limited to the country in which they and the practitioner are based, but not necessarily to the country where the issue of concern may have occurred. Challenges arise as a result of the increasing movement of healthcare professionals throughout the world, including the free movement of workers within the European Union. As a result, there is now closer working between regulators in different countries. For example, the GMC will routinely report any of their findings to overseas regulators where a doctor is known to have a link with them. GMC rules allow them to take action against a doctor on the basis of an adverse finding made by a regulator overseas. For reasons that are complex, overseas-trained doctors are more likely to face GMC sanctions than those trained in the UK. This is likely to be due to cultural differences and communication problems as well as other factors.

Further reading/resources

De Vries, H., Sanderson, P., Janta, B., Rabinovich, L., Archontakis, F., Ismail, S., Klautzer, L., Marjanovic, S., Patruni, B., Pru, S. and Tiessen, J. (2009) International comparison on ten medical regulatory systems. www.gmc-uk.org (accessed October 2016).

General Medical Council (2013) *Good Medical Practice.* www.gmc-uk.org (accessed October 2016).

Nursing and Midwifery Council (2015) The Code: Professional standards of practice and behaviour for nurses and midwives. www.nmc.org.uk (accessed October 2016).

Horsfall, S. (2014) Doctors who commit suicide while under GMC fitness to practice investigation. Internal Review. General Medical Council. www.gmc-uk.org (accessed October 2016).

Moszynski, P. (2007) GMC to look into higher number of complaints against overseas trained doctors. *British Medical Journal*, **335** (7615), 320.

Recommended Books, Articles and Websites

For students and teachers

Ballatt, J. and Campling, P. (2011) *Intelligent Kindness. Reforming the culture of healthcare*. RCPsych Publications, London.

Cooper, N. and Frain, J. (eds) (2017) *ABC of Clinical Communication*. Wiley, Oxford.

Creuss, R.L., Creuss, S.R. and Steinert, Y. (2016) *Teaching Medical Professionalism*. Cambridge University Press, Cambridge.

General Medical Council (2013) *Good Medical Practice*. General Medical Council, London.

General Medical Council (2016) *Professional Behaviour and Fitness to Practice – guidance for medical schools and their students*. General Medical Council, London.

Jones, P. (ed.) (2005) *Doctors as Patients*. Radcliffe, Oxford.

Kalanathi, P. (2016) *When Breath Becomes Air*. Bodley Head, London.

King's Fund (2008) *Understanding doctors: Harnessing professionalism*. King's Fund, London.

Levinson, W., Ginsburg, S., Hafferty, F.W. and Lucey, C.R. (2014) *Understanding Medical Professionalism*. McGraw-Hill Medical, New York.

Monrouxe, L.V. and Rees, C.E. (2017) *Healthcare professionalism. Improving practice through reflections on workplace dilemmas*. Wiley Blackwell, Oxford.

Nursing and Midwifery Council (2015) *The Code*. Nursing and Midwifery Council, London.

Spandorfer, J., Pohl, C.A., Rattner, S.L. and Nasca, T.J. (eds) (2009) *Professionalism in Medicine: A case-based guide for medical students*. Cambridge University Press, Cambridge.

Swanwick, T. and McKimm, J. (2017) *ABC of Clinical Leadership*. Wiley, Oxford.

Tate, P. and Tate, L. (2014) *The Doctor's Communication Handbook*. Radcliffe, London.

Rainham, D.C. (1996) *The Stress of Medicine*. ISBN 1-896181-17-1.

Thistlethwaite, J. and Spencer, J. (2008) *Professionalism in Medicine*. CRC Press, Boca Raton.

Thistlethwaite, J. and McKimm, J. (eds) (2015) *Health Care Professionalism at a Glance*. Wiley-Blackwell, Oxford.

Academic

ABIM Foundation, American Board of Internal Medicine, ACP-ASIM Foundation (2002) American College of Physicians-American Society of Internal Medicine, European Federation of Internal Medicine. Medical professionalism in the new millennium: A physician charter. *Annals of Internal Medicine*, **136** (3), 243–246.

Anagnostopoulos, F., Liolios, E., Persefonis, G., Slater, J., Kafetsios, K. and Niakas, D. (2012) Physician burnout and patient satisfaction with consultation in primary health care settings: evidence of relationships from a one-with-many design. *Journal of Clinical Psychology in Medical Settings*, **19** (4), 401–410.

Billings, M.E., Lazarus, M.E., Wenrich, M., Randall Curtis, J. and Engelberg, R.A. (2011) The effect of the hidden curriculum on resident burnout and cynicism. *Journal of Graduate Medical Education*. dx.dol.org/10-4300/JGME-D-11-00044.1

Bourne, T., Vanderhaegan, J., Vranken, R., Wynants, L., De Cock, B., Peters, M. *et al.* (2016) Doctors' experiences and their perception of complaints processes in the UK: an analysis of qualitative survey data. *British Medical Journal Open*. DOI: 10.1136/bmjopen-2016-011711 (accessed April 2017).

Bourne, T., Wynants, L., Peters, M., Van Audenhove, C., Timmerman, A., Van Caister, B. *et al.* (2015) The impact of complaints procedures on the welfare, health and clinical practice of 7926 doctors in the UK: a cross-sectional survey. *British Medical Journal Open*, **4**, e006687 (accessed April 2017).

Brazeau, C.M.L.R., Schroeder, R., Rovi, S. *et al.* (2010) Relationships between medical student burnout, empathy, and professionalism climate. *Academic Medicine*, **85**, S33–S36.

British Medical Association (2004) *Safe Handover, Safe Patients. Guidance on Clinical Handover for Clinicians and Managers*. British Medical Association, London.

Bryden, P., Ginsburg, S. and Kurabi, B. (2010) Professing professionalism: are we our own worst enemy? Faculty members' experiences of teaching and evaluating professionalism in medical education at one medical school. *Academic Medicine*, **85**, 1025–1034.

Casey, D. and Choong, K.A. (2016) Suicide whilst under GMC's fitness to practise investigation: were those deaths preventable? *Journal of Forensic Legal Medicine*, **37**, 22–27.

Cecil, J., McHale, C., Hart, J. and Laidlaw, A. (2014) Behaviour and burnout in medical students. *Medical Education Online*, **19**, 10.3402/meo.v19.25209. DOI:10.3402/meo.v19.25209.

Chandratilake, M., McAleer, S., Gibson, J. *et al.* (2010) Medical professionalism: what does the public think? *Clinical Medicine*, **10**, 364–369.

Coverdale, J.H., Balon, R. and Roberts, L.W. (2009) Mistreatment of trainees: verbal abuse and other bullying behaviours. *Academic Psychiatry*, **33**, 269–273.

Cruess, S.R. and Cruess, R.L. (2000) Professionalism: a contract between medicine and society. *Canadian Medical Association Journal*, **162**, 668–669.

ABC of Clinical Professionalism, First Edition. Edited by Nicola Cooper, Anna Frain and John Frain.
© 2018 John Wiley & Sons Ltd. Published 2018 by John Wiley & Sons Ltd.

Dyrbye, L.N., Massie, F.S., Eacker, A. *et al.* (2010) Relationship between burnout and professional conduct and attitudes among US medical students. *Journal of the American Medical Association,* **304,** 1173–1180.

Dyrbye, L.N., Thomas, M.R., Harper, W. *et al.* (2009) The learning environment and medical student burnout: a multicenter study. *Medical Education,* **43,** 274–282.

Francis, R. (2013) Report of the Mid Staffordshire NHS Foundation Trust Public Inquiry: Executive summary.

Ginsburg, S. and Lingard, L. (2011) 'Is that normal?' Pre-clerkship students' approaches to professional dilemmas. *Medical Education,* **45,** 362–371.

Hafferty, F.W. (1998) Beyond curriculum reform: confronting medicine's hidden curriculum. *Academic Medicine,* **73,** 403–407.

Hilton, S.R. and Slotnick, H.B. (2005) Proto-professionalism: how professionalism occurs across the continuum of medical education. *Medical Education,* **39,** 58–65.

Hojat, M., Vergare, M.J., Maxwell, K. *et al.* (2009) The devil is in the third year: a longitudinal study of erosion of empathy in medical school. *Academic Medicine,* **84,** 1182–1191.

Humprey, H.J., Smith, K., Reddy, S., Scott, D., Madara, J.L. and Arora, V.M. (2007) Promoting an environment of professionalism: the University of Chicago "roadmap". *Academic Medicine,* **82** (11), 1098–1107.

Iverson, A., Rushforth, B. and Forrest, K. (2009) How to handle stress and look after yourself. *British Medical Journal,* **338,** b1368.

Karnieli-Miller, O., Vu, R., Frankel, R.M. *et al.* (2011) Which experiences in the hidden curriculum teach students about professionalism? *Academic Medicine,* **86,** 369–377.

Landman, M., Shelton, J. and Kauffmann, R.M. (2010) Guidelines for maintaining a professional compass in the era of social networking. *Journal of Surgery,* **67,** 381–386.

Lee, K.L. and Ho, M.J. (2011) Online social networking versus medical professionalism. *Medical Education,* **45,** 523.

Mostaghimi, A. and Crotty, B.H. (2011) Professionalism in the digital age. *Annals of Internal Medicine,* **154,** 560–562.

Papadakis, M.A., Teherani, A., Banach, M.A, *et al.* (2005) Disciplinary action by medical boards and prior behaviour in medical school. *New England Journal of Medicine,* **353,** 2673–2682.

Riskin, A., Erez, A., Foulk, T.A. *et al.* (2015) The impact of rudeness on medical team performance: a randomised trial. *Pediatrics,* **136** (3), 487–495.

Shanafelt, T.D., Bradley, K.A., Wipf, J.E. and Back, A.L. (2002) Burnout and self-reported patient care in an internal medicine residency program. *Annals of Internal Medicine,* **136,** 358–367.

Shanafelt, T.D., Balch, C.M., Bechamps, G. *et al.* (2010) Burnout and medical errors among American surgeons. *Annals of Surgery,* **251** (6), 995–1000.

Skelton, J.R., Wearn, A.M. and Hobbs, F.D.R. (2002) 'I' and 'We': a concordancing analysis of how doctors and patients use first person pronouns in primary care consultations. *Family Practice,* **19,** 484–488.

Sox, C.H. (2007) The ethical foundations of professionalism: a sociologic history. *Chest,* **131,** 1532–1540.

Todhunter, S., Cruess, S.R., Cruess, R.L. *et al.* (2011) Developing and piloting a form for student assessment of faculty professionalism. *Advances in Health Science and Education,* **16,** 223–238.

Passi, V. and Johnson, N. (2016) The impact of positive doctor role modelling. *Medical Teacher.* DOI: 10.3109/0142159X.2016.1170780 (accessed April 2014).

Wear, D., Aultman, J.M., Zarconi, J. and Varley, J.D. (2009) Derogatory and cynical humour directed towards patients: views of residents and attending doctors. *Medical Education,* **43,** 34–41.

Wessely, A. and Gerada, C. (2013) When doctors need treatment: an anthropological approach to why doctors make bad patients. *British Medical Journal Careers* http://careers.bmj.com/careers/advice/view-article.html?id=20015402 (accessed April 2014).

West, C.P., Dyrbye, L.N., Erwin, P.J. and Shanafelt, T.D. (2016) Interventions to prevent and reduce physician burnout: a systematic review and meta-analysis. *Lancet,* **388,** 2272–2281.

Yates, J. and James, D. (2010) Risk factors at medical school for subsequent professional misconduct: multicentre retrospective case-control study. *British Medical Journal,* **340,** 2040.

Websites (all accessed April 2017)

American Medical Association: www.ama-assn.org.

The Canadian Interprofessional Health Collaborative www.cihc.ca.

Choosing wisely campaign: www.choosingwisely.co.uk.

Clinical Human Factors Group: http://chfg.org.

General Medical Council (UK): www.gmc-uk.org.

Health and Care Professions Council (UK) www.hcpc-uk.org.

Just a routine operation: https://www.youtube.com/watch?v=JzlvgtPIof4.

NHS Practitioner Health Programme: http://php.nhs.uk.

Nursing and Midwifery Council (UK): www.nmc.org.uk.

Royal Australian College of General Practitioners: www.racgp.org.

ephysicianhealth.com (accessed August 2017).

Index

ABC of Clinical Professionalism, First Edition. Edited by Nicola Cooper, Anna Frain and John Frain.
© 2018 John Wiley & Sons Ltd. Published 2018 by John Wiley & Sons Ltd.